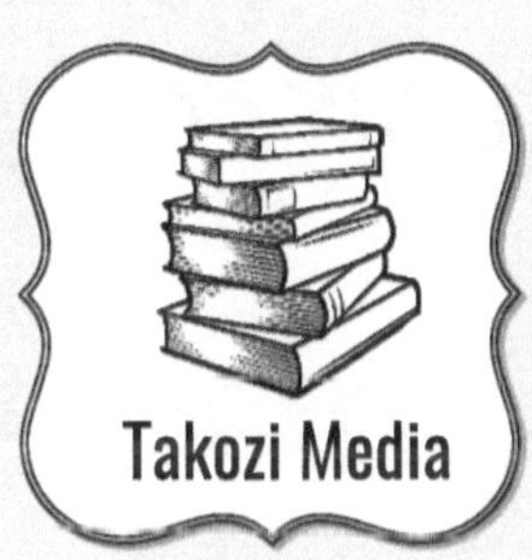

Takozi Media

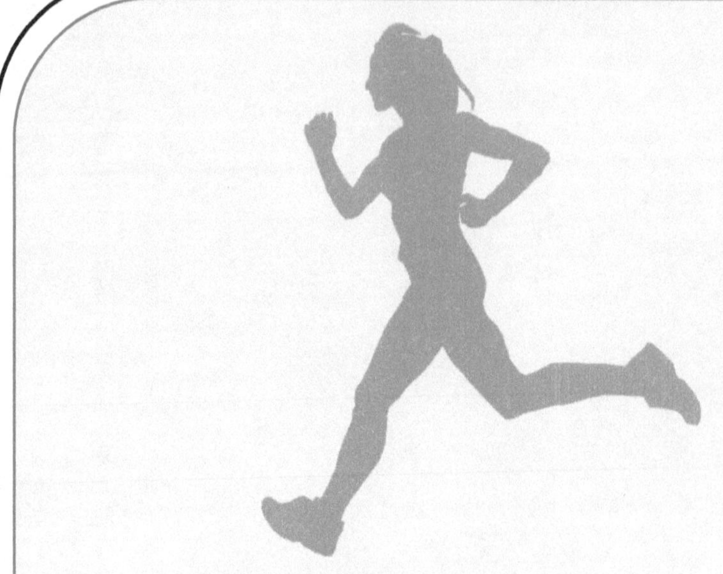

This Book Belongs To:

....

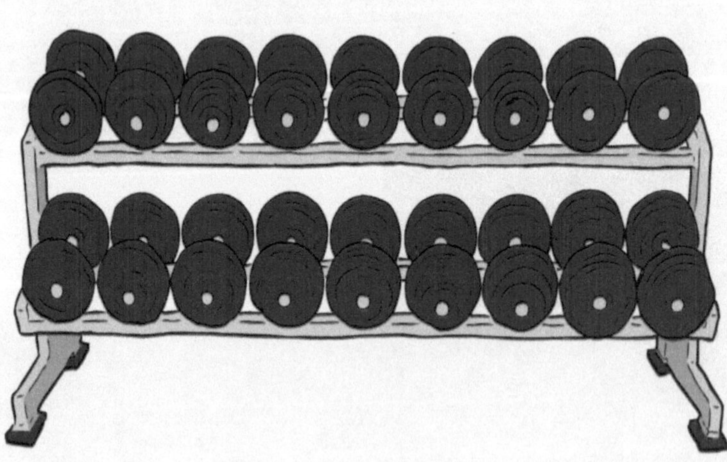

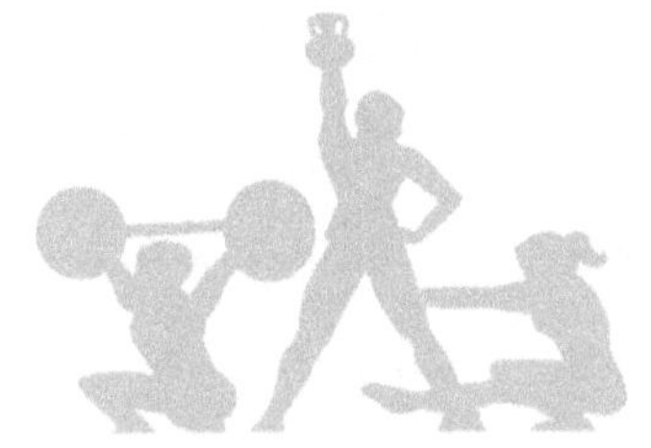

Name: ....
Date: ....
Time: ....

Warm-Up

ACTIVITY	TIME/REPS	DONE

 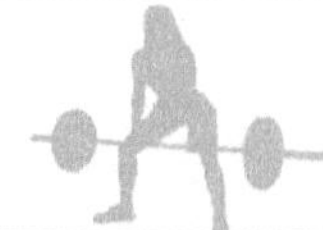 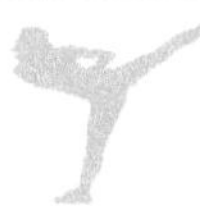 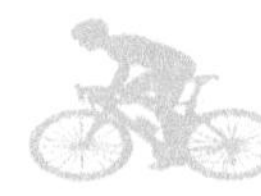

Cardio

ACTIVITY	DISTANCE	TIME	DONE

Weight Training

EXERCISE	SET ONE WEIGHT/REPS	SET TWO WEIGHT/REPS	SET THREE WEIGHT/REPS

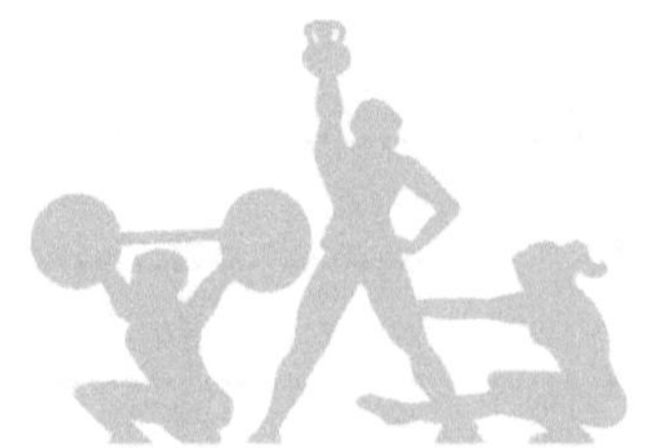

Name: ……………………….

Date: ……………………….

Time: ……………………….

Warm-Up

ACTIVITY	TIME/REPS	DONE

 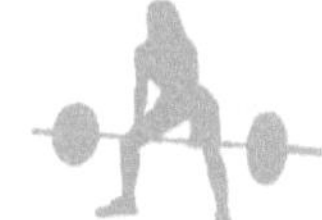 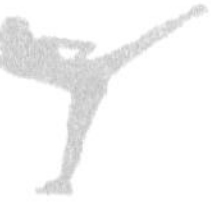 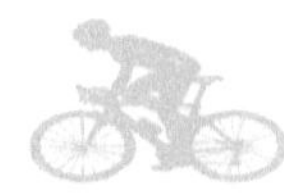

Cardio

ACTIVITY	DISTANCE	TIME	DONE

Weight Training

EXERCISE	SET ONE WEIGHT/REPS	SET TWO WEIGHT/REPS	SET THREE WEIGHT/REPS

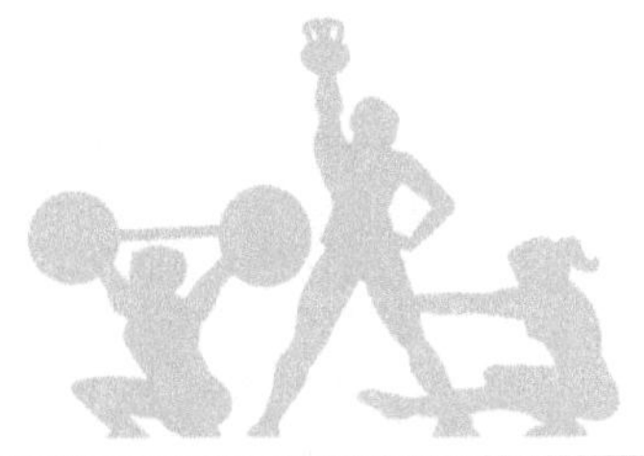

Name: ....

Date: ....

Time: ....

Warm-Up

ACTIVITY	TIME/REPS	DONE

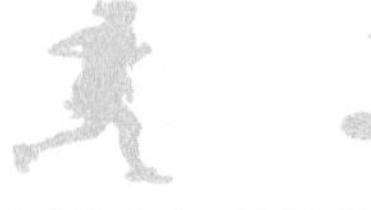 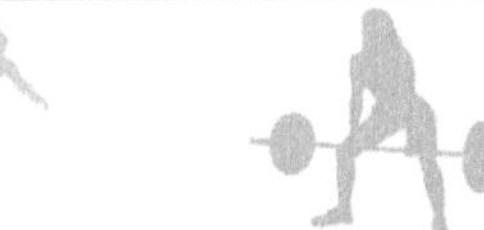 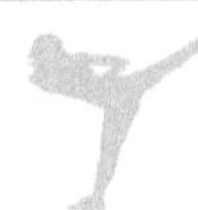 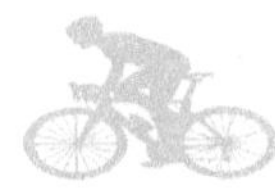

Cardio

ACTIVITY	DISTANCE	TIME	DONE

Weight Training

EXERCISE	SET ONE WEIGHT/REPS	SET TWO WEIGHT/REPS	SET THREE WEIGHT/REPS

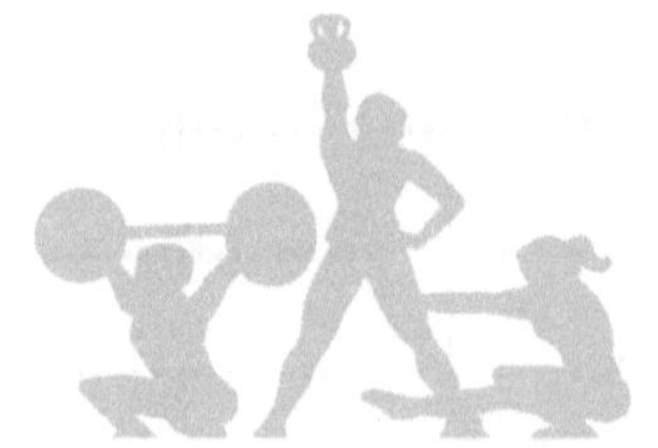

Name: ....

Date: ....

Time: ....

Warm-Up

ACTIVITY	TIME/REPS	DONE

 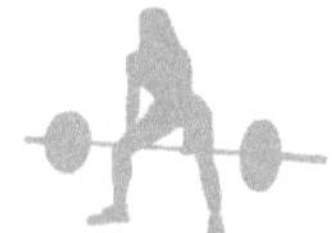 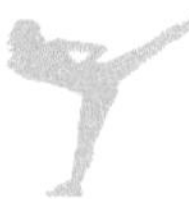 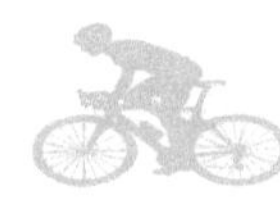

Cardio

ACTIVITY	DISTANCE	TIME	DONE

Weight Training

EXERCISE	SET ONE WEIGHT/REPS	SET TWO WEIGHT/REPS	SET THREE WEIGHT/REPS

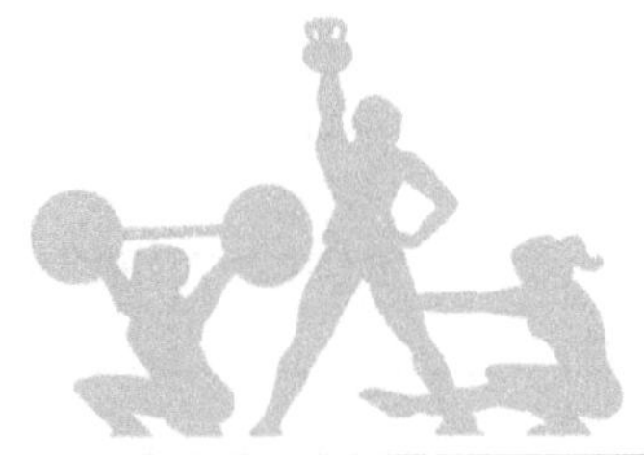

Name: ....

Date: ....

Time: ....

Warm-Up

ACTIVITY	TIME/REPS	DONE

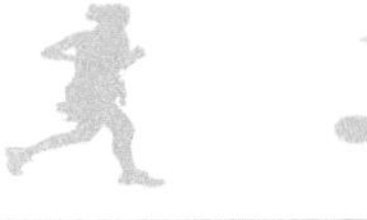 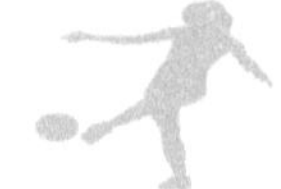 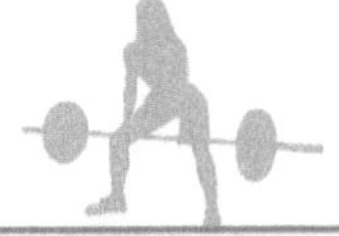 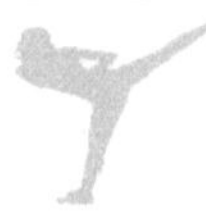 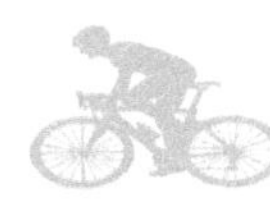

Cardio

ACTIVITY	DISTANCE	TIME	DONE

Weight Training

EXERCISE	SET ONE WEIGHT/REPS	SET TWO WEIGHT/REPS	SET THREE WEIGHT/REPS

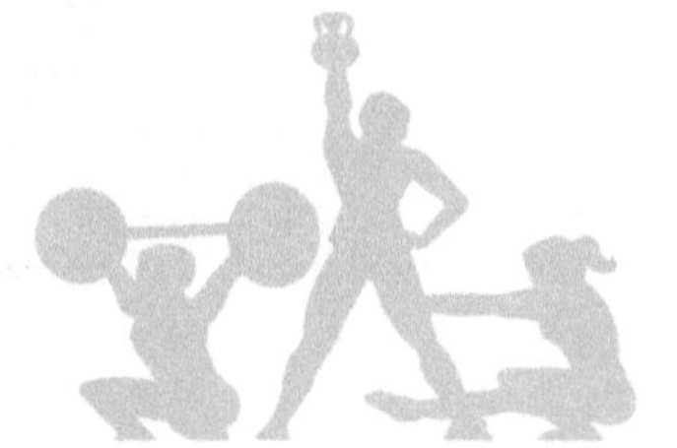

Name: ....

Date: ....

Time: ....

Warm-Up

ACTIVITY	TIME/REPS	DONE

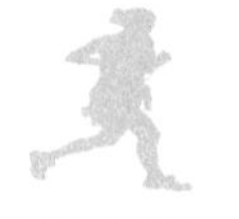 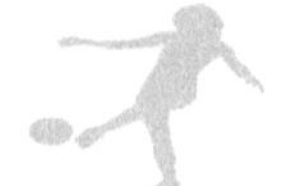 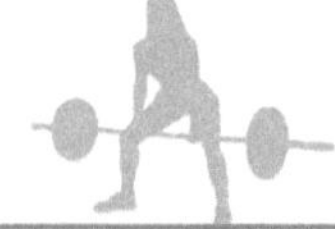 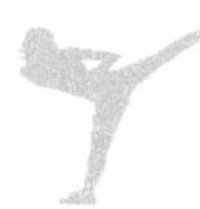 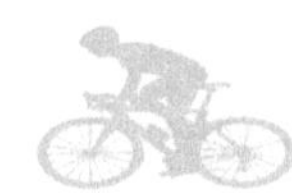

Cardio

ACTIVITY	DISTANCE	TIME	DONE

Weight Training

EXERCISE	SET ONE WEIGHT/REPS	SET TWO WEIGHT/REPS	SET THREE WEIGHT/REPS

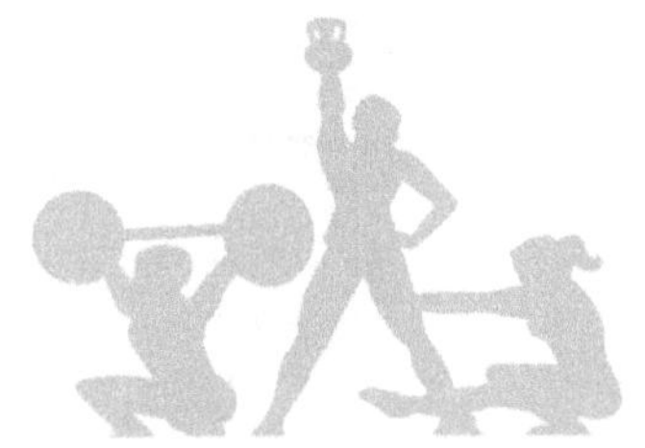

Name: ....

Date: ....

Time: ....

Warm-Up

ACTIVITY	TIME/REPS	DONE

  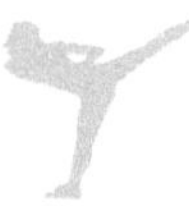 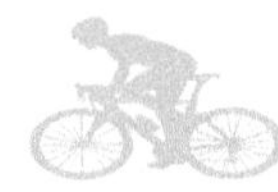

Cardio

ACTIVITY	DISTANCE	TIME	DONE

Weight Training

EXERCISE	SET ONE WEIGHT/REPS	SET TWO WEIGHT/REPS	SET THREE WEIGHT/REPS

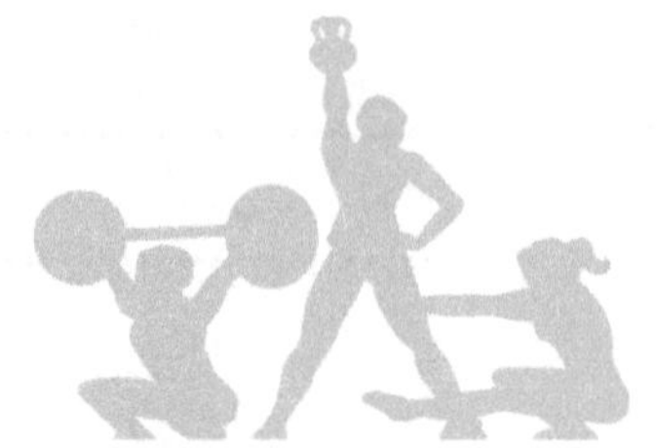

Name: ....

Date: ....

Time: ....

Warm-Up

ACTIVITY	TIME/REPS	DONE

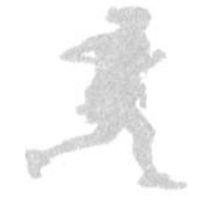  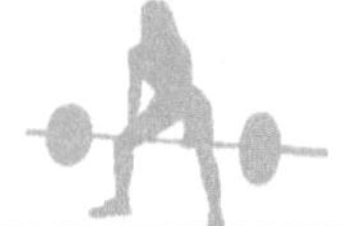 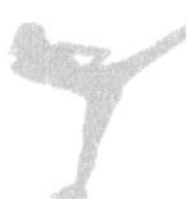 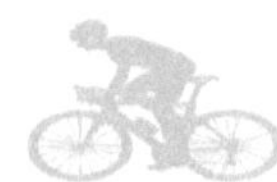

Cardio

ACTIVITY	DISTANCE	TIME	DONE

Weight Training

EXERCISE	SET ONE WEIGHT/REPS	SET TWO WEIGHT/REPS	SET THREE WEIGHT/REPS

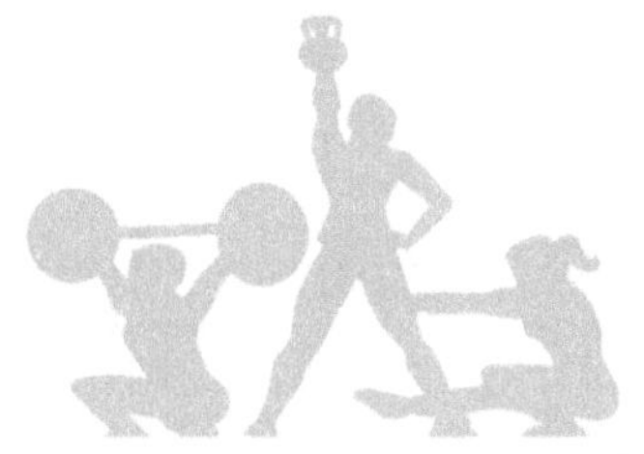

Name: …………………………

Date: …………………………

Time: …………………………

Warm-Up

ACTIVITY	TIME/REPS	DONE

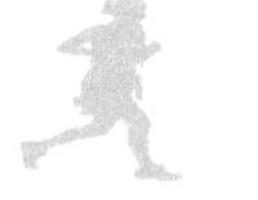 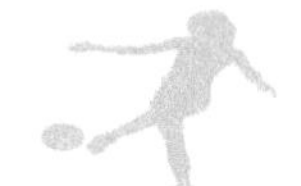 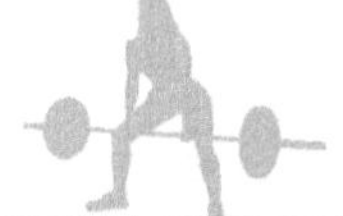 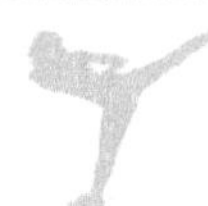 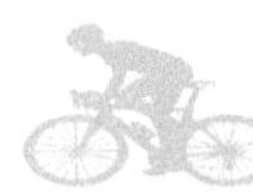

Cardio

ACTIVITY	DISTANCE	TIME	DONE

Weight Training

EXERCISE	SET ONE WEIGHT/REPS	SET TWO WEIGHT/REPS	SET THREE WEIGHT/REPS

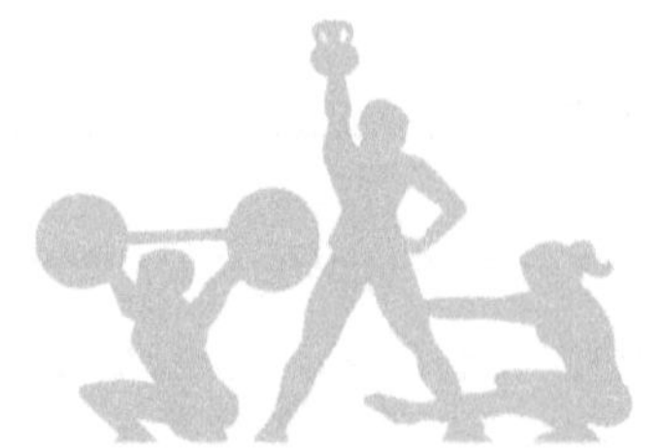

Name: ....

Date: ....

Time: ....

Warm-Up

ACTIVITY	TIME/REPS	DONE

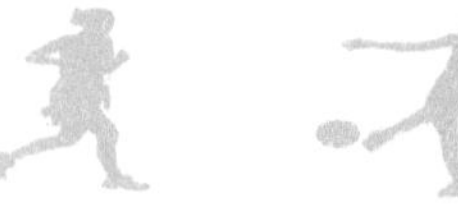 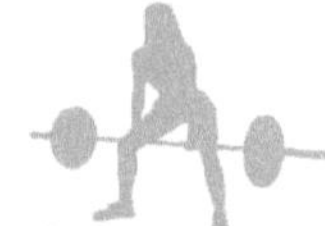 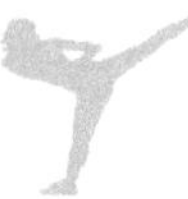 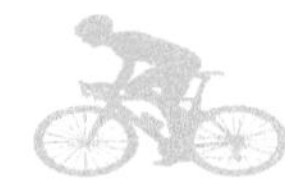

Cardio

ACTIVITY	DISTANCE	TIME	DONE

Weight Training

EXERCISE	SET ONE WEIGHT/REPS	SET TWO WEIGHT/REPS	SET THREE WEIGHT/REPS

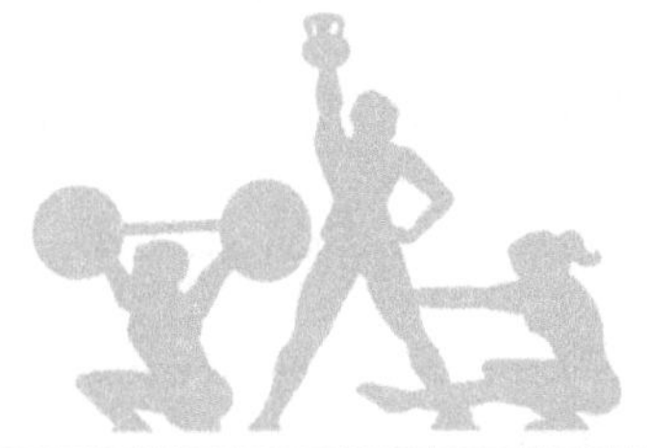

Warm-Up

ACTIVITY	TIME/REPS	DONE

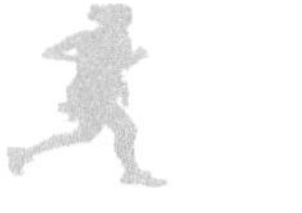 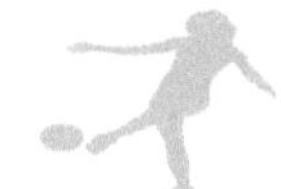 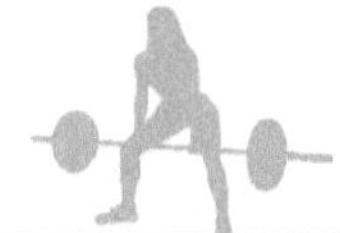 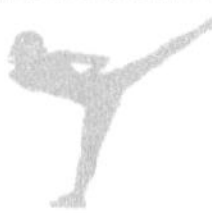 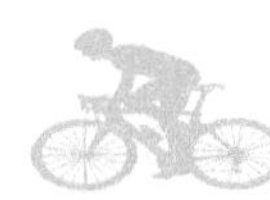

Cardio

ACTIVITY	DISTANCE	TIME	DONE

Weight Training

EXERCISE	SET ONE WEIGHT/REPS	SET TWO WEIGHT/REPS	SET THREE WEIGHT/REPS

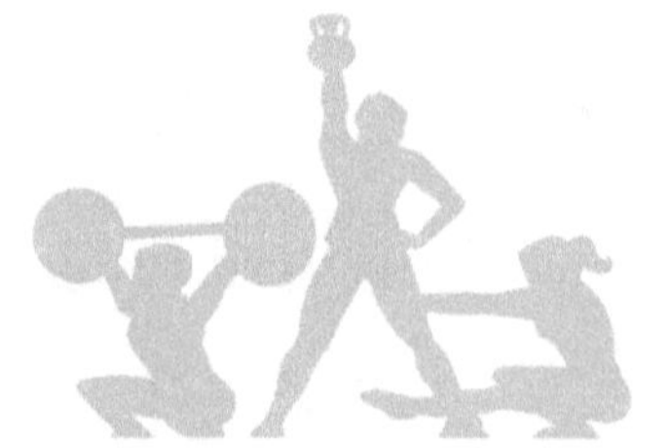

Name: ....

Date: ....

Time: ....

Warm-Up

ACTIVITY	TIME/REPS	DONE

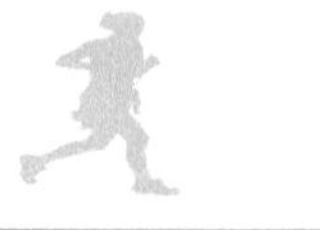 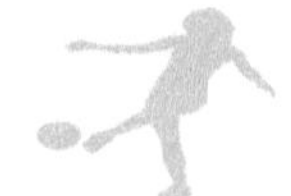 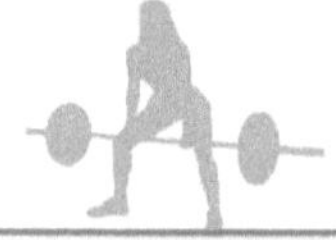 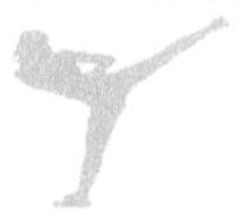 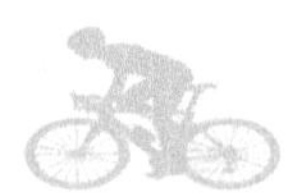

Cardio

ACTIVITY	DISTANCE	TIME	DONE

Weight Training

EXERCISE	SET ONE WEIGHT/REPS	SET TWO WEIGHT/REPS	SET THREE WEIGHT/REPS

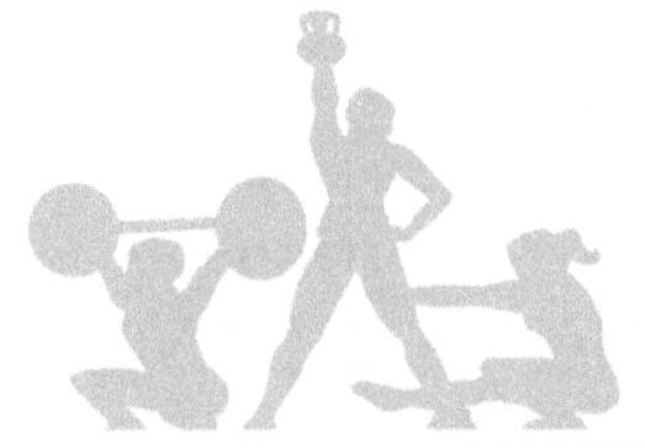

Name: ....

Date: ....

Time: ....

Warm-Up

ACTIVITY	TIME/REPS	DONE

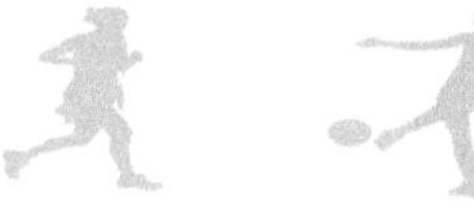 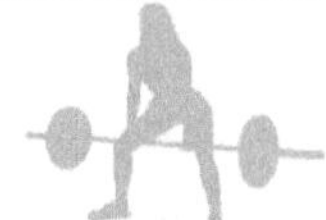 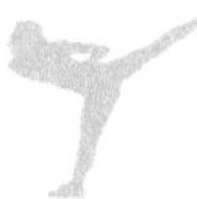 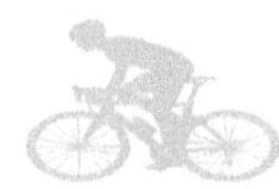

Cardio

ACTIVITY	DISTANCE	TIME	DONE

Weight Training

EXERCISE	SET ONE WEIGHT/REPS	SET TWO WEIGHT/REPS	SET THREE WEIGHT/REPS

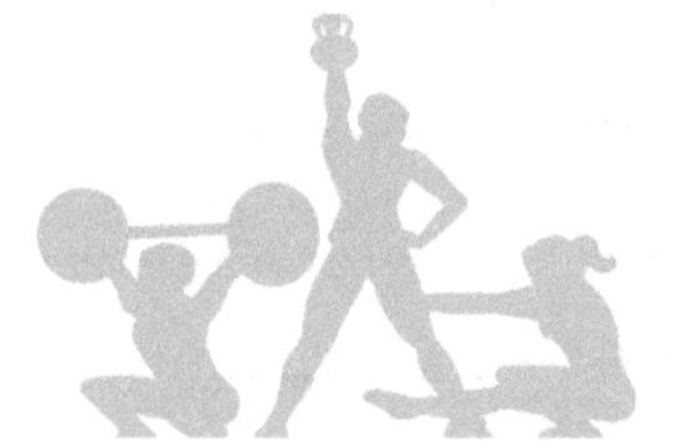

Warm-Up

ACTIVITY	TIME/REPS	DONE

 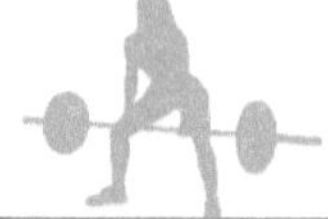 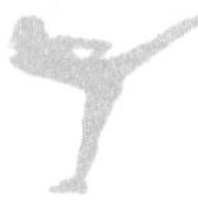 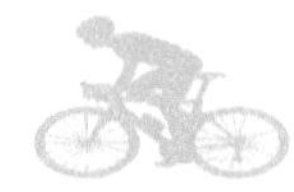

Cardio

ACTIVITY	DISTANCE	TIME	DONE

Weight Training

EXERCISE	SET ONE WEIGHT/REPS	SET TWO WEIGHT/REPS	SET THREE WEIGHT/REPS

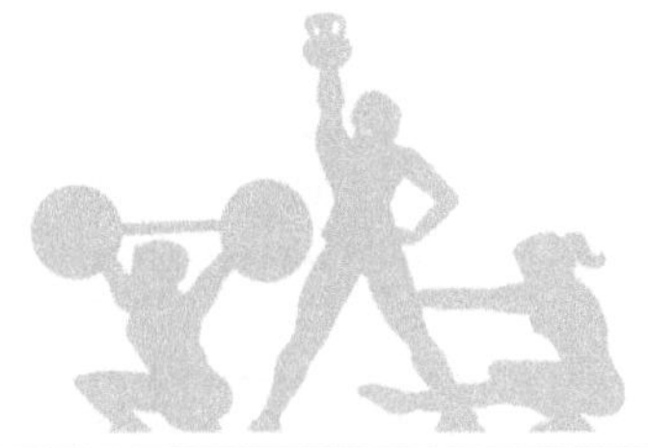

Warm-Up

ACTIVITY	TIME/REPS	DONE

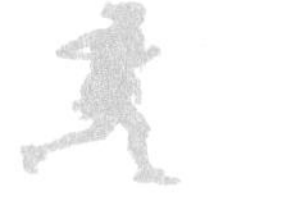   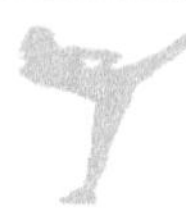 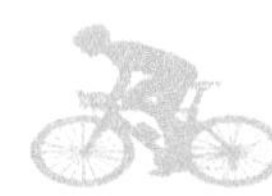

Cardio

ACTIVITY	DISTANCE	TIME	DONE

Weight Training

EXERCISE	SET ONE WEIGHT/REPS	SET TWO WEIGHT/REPS	SET THREE WEIGHT/REPS

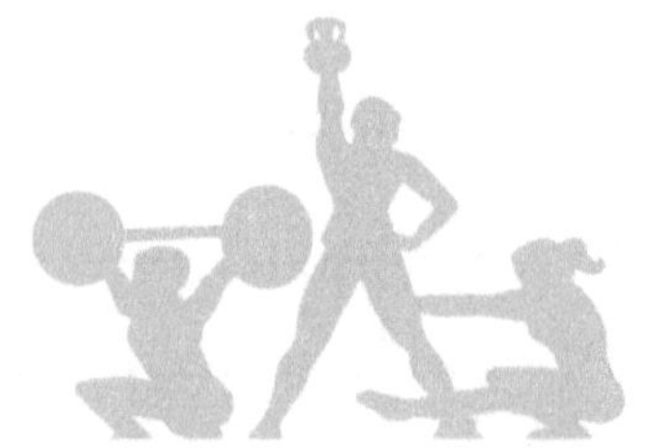

Name: ……………………………

Date: ……………………………

Time: ……………………………

Warm-Up

ACTIVITY	TIME/REPS	DONE

 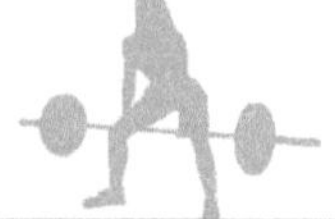 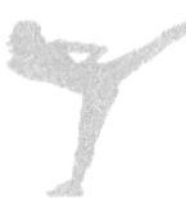 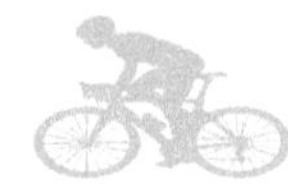

Cardio

ACTIVITY	DISTANCE	TIME	DONE

Weight Training

EXERCISE	SET ONE WEIGHT/REPS	SET TWO WEIGHT/REPS	SET THREE WEIGHT/REPS

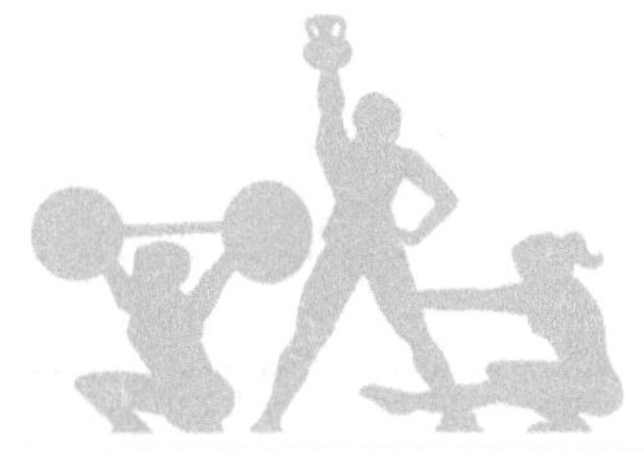

Name: ....

Date: ....

Time: ....

Warm-Up

ACTIVITY	TIME/REPS	DONE

 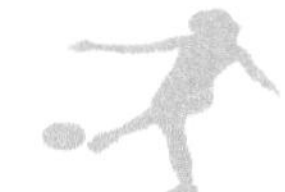 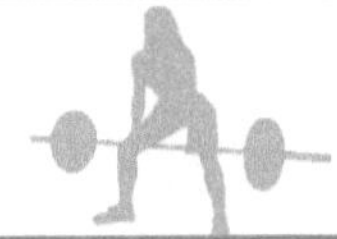 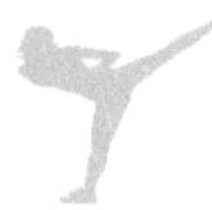 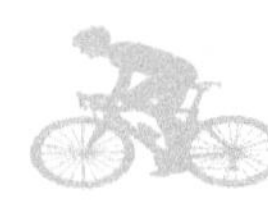

Cardio

ACTIVITY	DISTANCE	TIME	DONE

Weight Training

EXERCISE	SET ONE WEIGHT/REPS	SET TWO WEIGHT/REPS	SET THREE WEIGHT/REPS

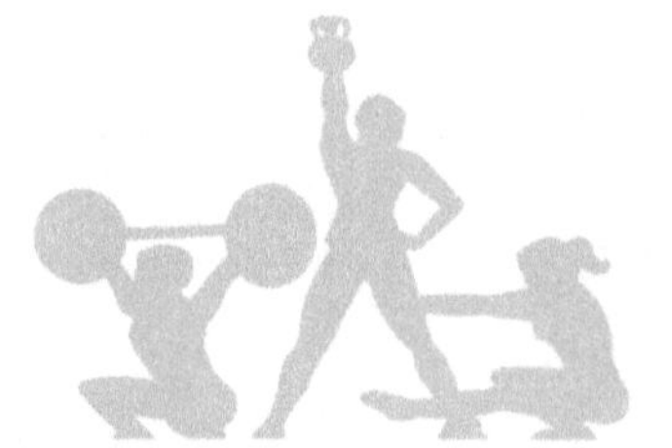

Name: ....

Date: ....

Time: ....

Warm-Up

ACTIVITY	TIME/REPS	DONE

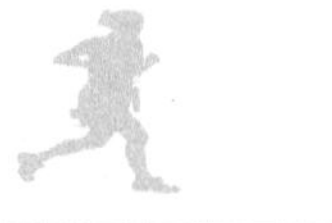 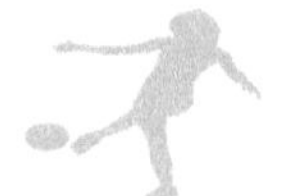 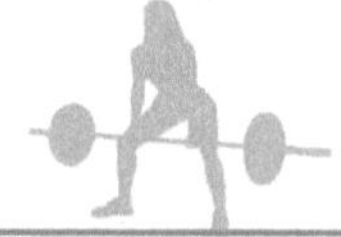 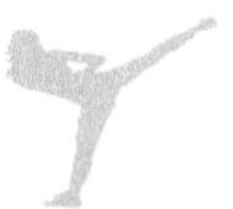 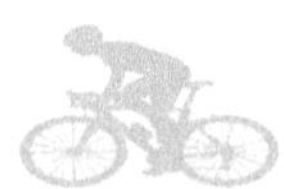

Cardio

ACTIVITY	DISTANCE	TIME	DONE

Weight Training

EXERCISE	SET ONE WEIGHT/REPS	SET TWO WEIGHT/REPS	SET THREE WEIGHT/REPS

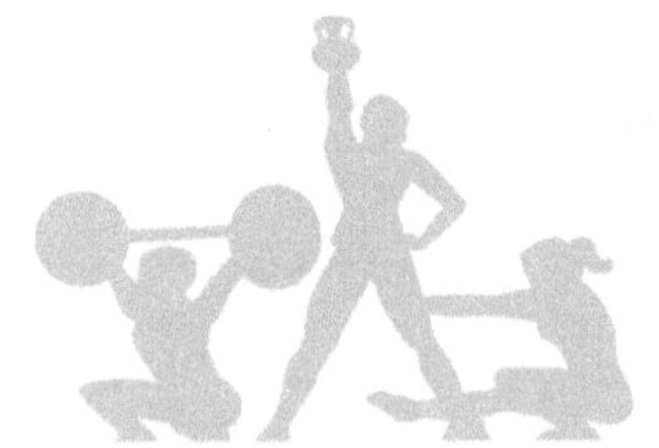

Name: ………………………………

Date: ………………………………

Time: ………………………………

Warm-Up

ACTIVITY	TIME/REPS	DONE

 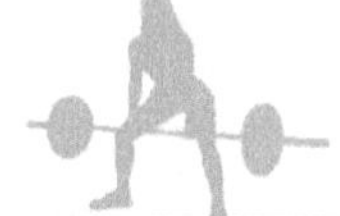 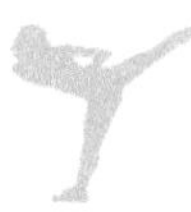 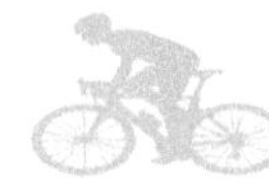

Cardio

ACTIVITY	DISTANCE	TIME	DONE

Weight Training

EXERCISE	SET ONE WEIGHT/REPS	SET TWO WEIGHT/REPS	SET THREE WEIGHT/REPS

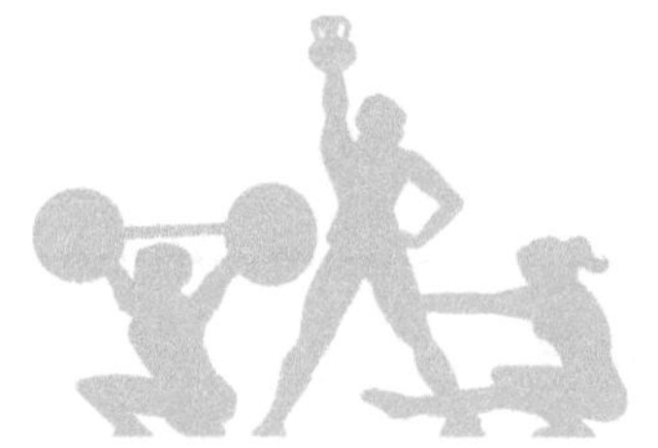

Name: ……………………………

Date: ……………………………

Time: ……………………………

Warm-Up

ACTIVITY	TIME/REPS	DONE

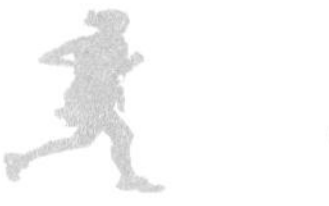 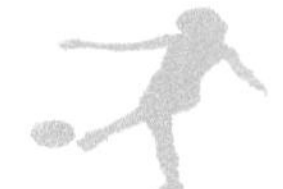 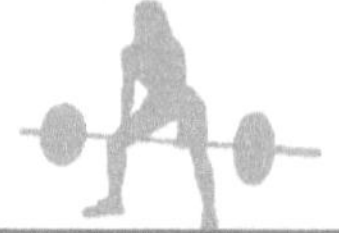 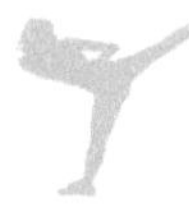 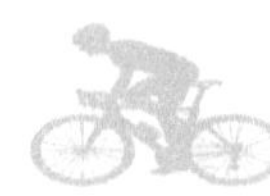

Cardio

ACTIVITY	DISTANCE	TIME	DONE

Weight Training

EXERCISE	SET ONE WEIGHT/REPS	SET TWO WEIGHT/REPS	SET THREE WEIGHT/REPS

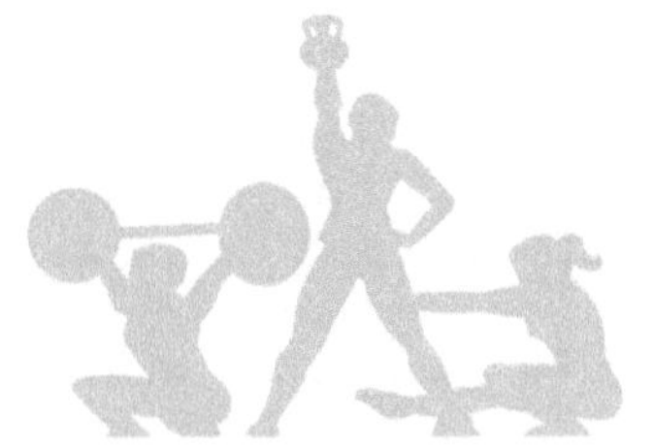

Name: ....

Date: ....

Time: ....

Warm-Up

ACTIVITY	TIME/REPS	DONE

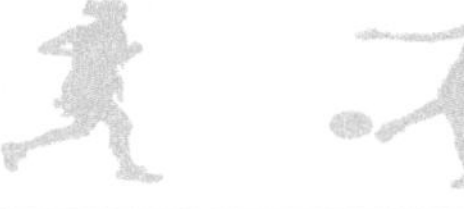 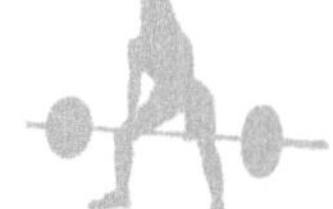 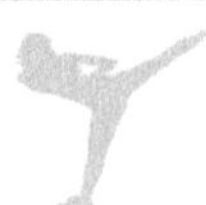 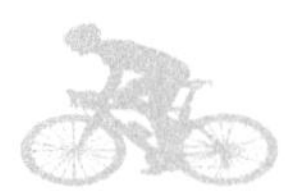

Cardio

ACTIVITY	DISTANCE	TIME	DONE

Weight Training

EXERCISE	SET ONE WEIGHT/REPS	SET TWO WEIGHT/REPS	SET THREE WEIGHT/REPS

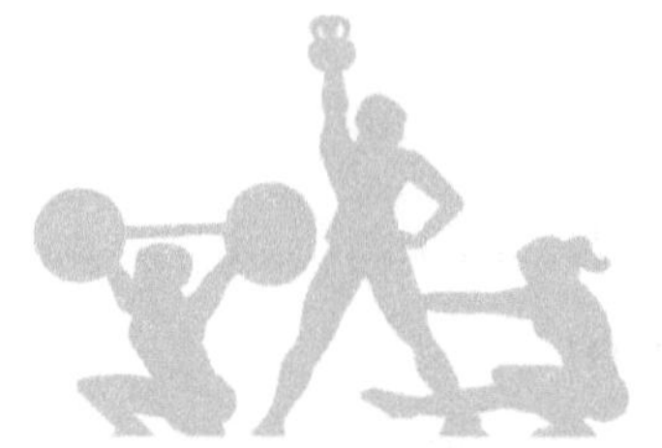

Name: ....

Date: ....

Time: ....

Warm-Up

ACTIVITY	TIME/REPS	DONE

 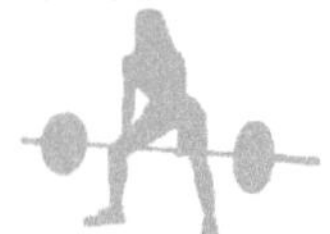  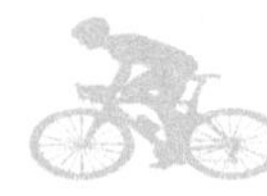

Cardio

ACTIVITY	DISTANCE	TIME	DONE

Weight Training

EXERCISE	SET ONE WEIGHT/REPS	SET TWO WEIGHT/REPS	SET THREE WEIGHT/REPS

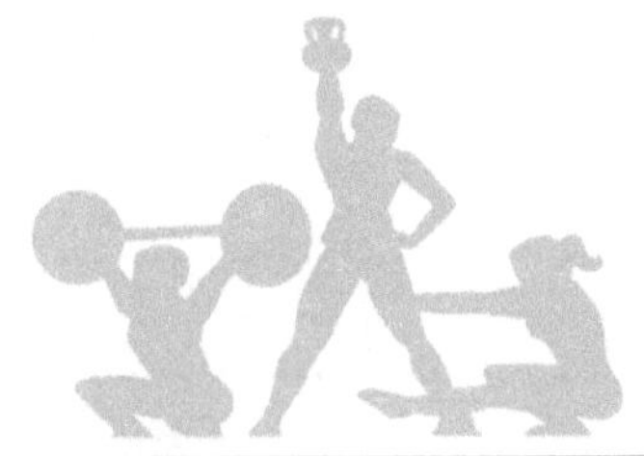

Name: ....

Date: ....

Time: ....

Warm-Up

ACTIVITY	TIME/REPS	DONE

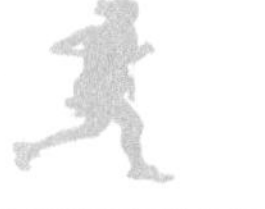 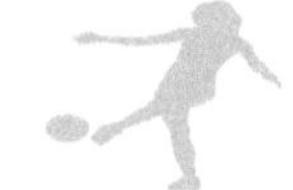 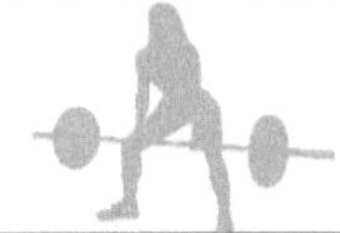 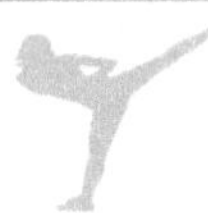 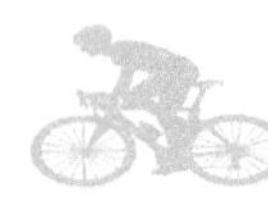

Cardio

ACTIVITY	DISTANCE	TIME	DONE

Weight Training

EXERCISE	SET ONE WEIGHT/REPS	SET TWO WEIGHT/REPS	SET THREE WEIGHT/REPS

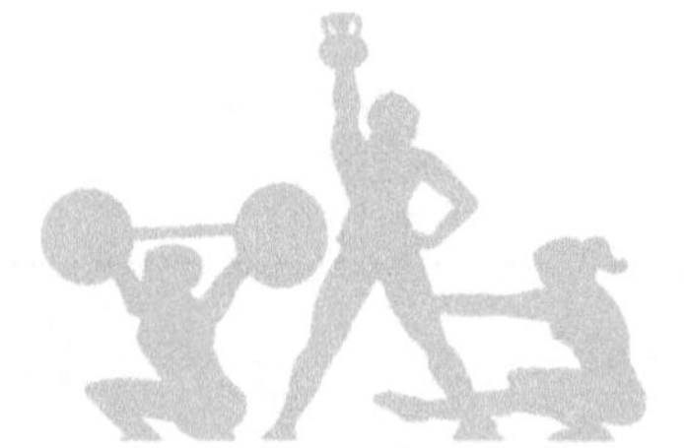

Name: ....

Date: ....

Time: ....

Warm-Up

ACTIVITY	TIME/REPS	DONE

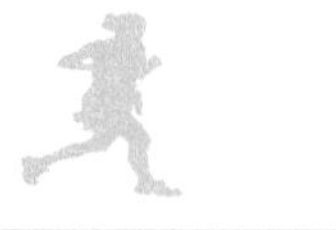  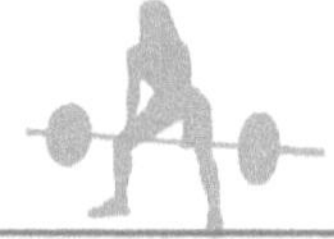 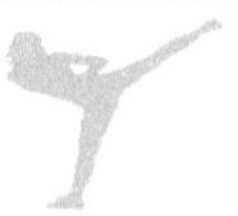 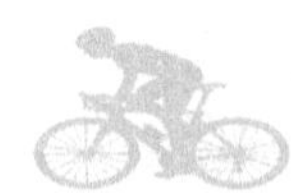

Cardio

ACTIVITY	DISTANCE	TIME	DONE

Weight Training

EXERCISE	SET ONE WEIGHT/REPS	SET TWO WEIGHT/REPS	SET THREE WEIGHT/REPS

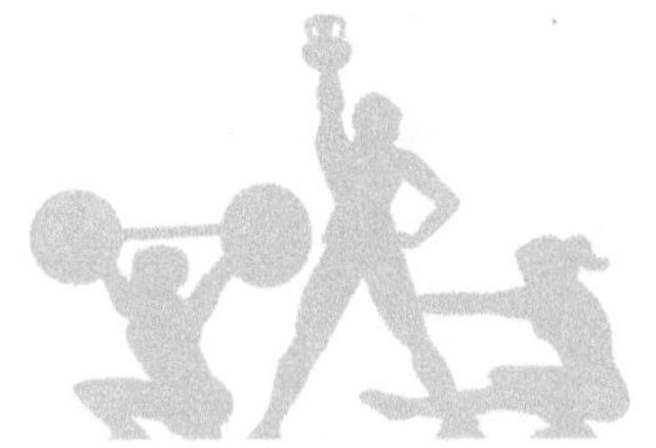

Name: …………………………

Date: …………………………

Time: …………………………

Warm-Up

ACTIVITY	TIME/REPS	DONE

 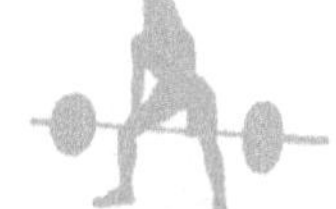 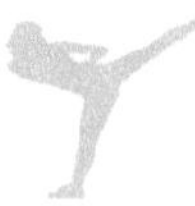 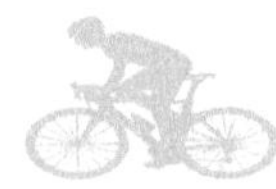

Cardio

ACTIVITY	DISTANCE	TIME	DONE

Weight Training

EXERCISE	SET ONE WEIGHT/REPS	SET TWO WEIGHT/REPS	SET THREE WEIGHT/REPS

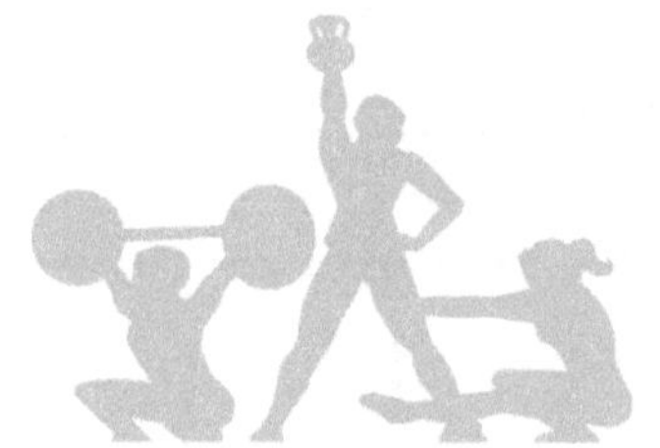

Name: ....

Date: ....

Time: ....

Warm-Up

ACTIVITY	TIME/REPS	DONE

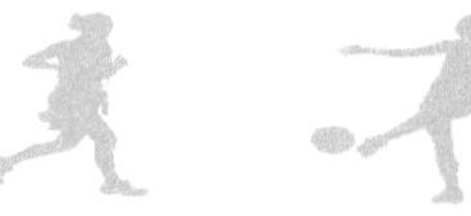 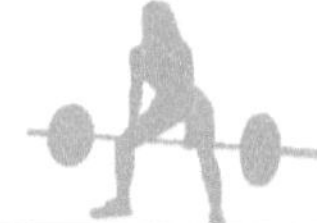 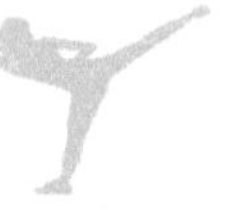 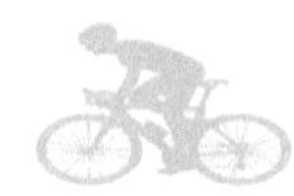

Cardio

ACTIVITY	DISTANCE	TIME	DONE

Weight Training

EXERCISE	SET ONE WEIGHT/REPS	SET TWO WEIGHT/REPS	SET THREE WEIGHT/REPS

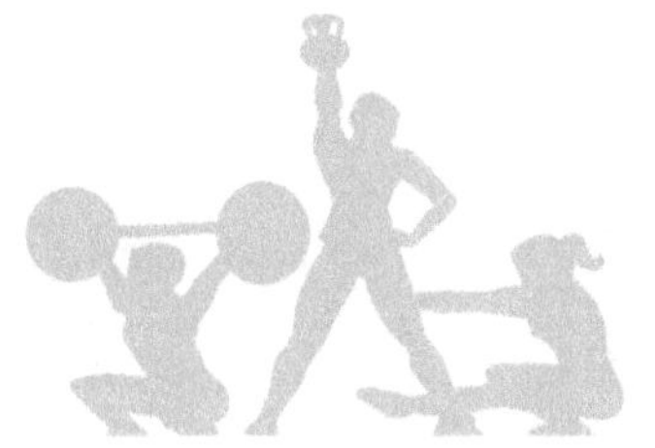

Name: ……………………………

Date: ……………………………

Time: ……………………………

Warm-Up

ACTIVITY	TIME/REPS	DONE

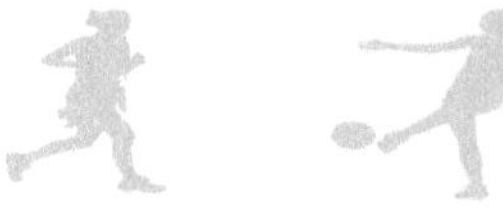 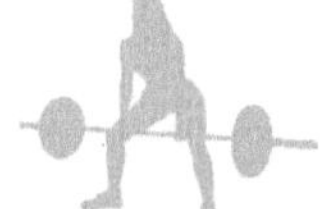 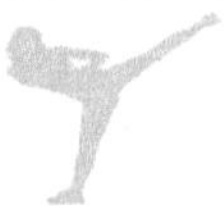 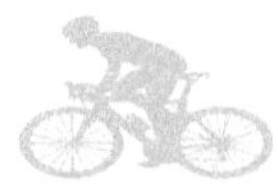

Cardio

ACTIVITY	DISTANCE	TIME	DONE

Weight Training

EXERCISE	SET ONE WEIGHT/REPS	SET TWO WEIGHT/REPS	SET THREE WEIGHT/REPS

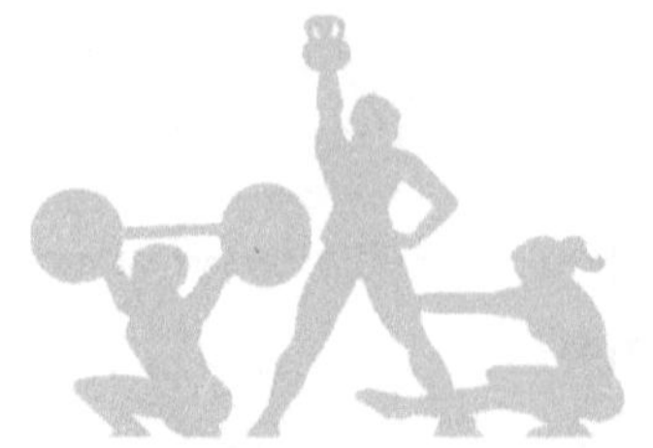

Name: ....

Date: ....

Time: ....

Warm-Up

ACTIVITY	TIME/REPS	DONE

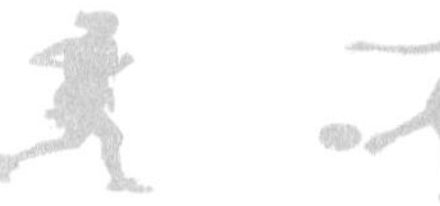 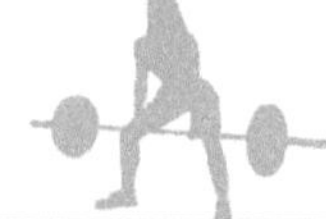 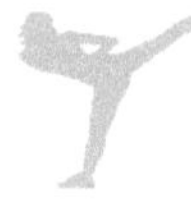 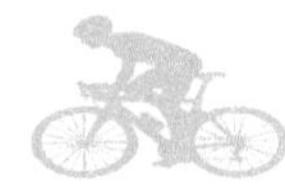

Cardio

ACTIVITY	DISTANCE	TIME	DONE

Weight Training

EXERCISE	SET ONE WEIGHT/REPS	SET TWO WEIGHT/REPS	SET THREE WEIGHT/REPS

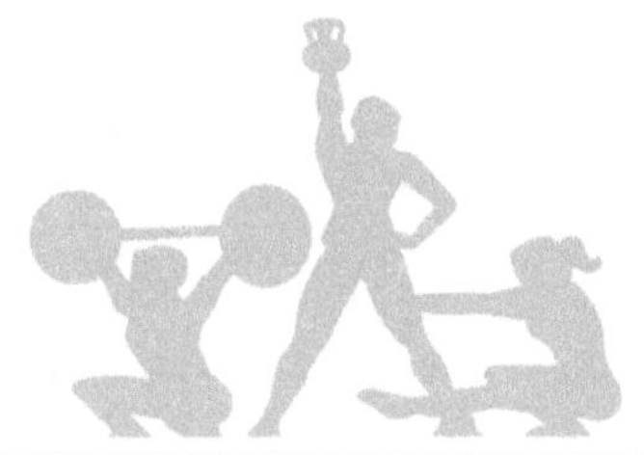

Warm-Up

ACTIVITY	TIME/REPS	DONE

 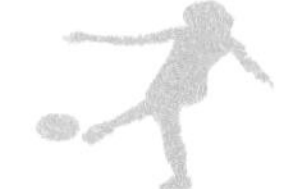 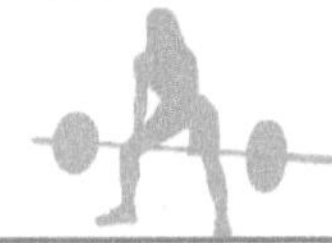 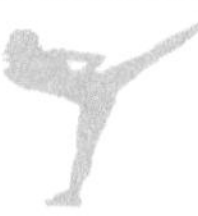 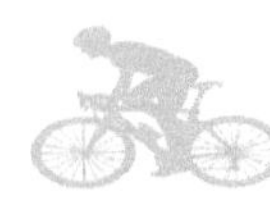

Cardio

ACTIVITY	DISTANCE	TIME	DONE

Weight Training

EXERCISE	SET ONE WEIGHT/REPS	SET TWO WEIGHT/REPS	SET THREE WEIGHT/REPS

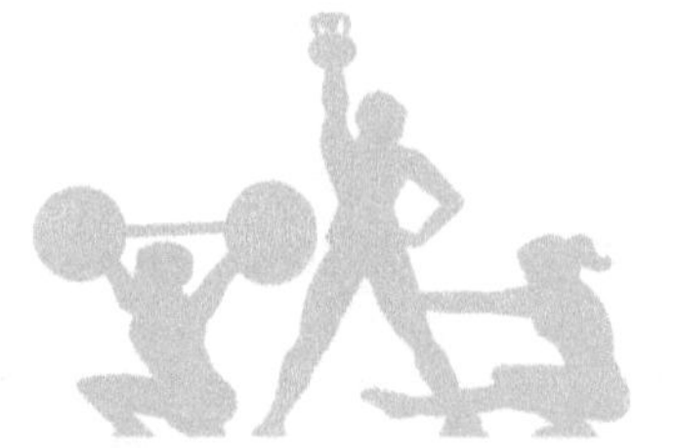

Name: ....

Date: ....

Time: ....

Warm-Up

ACTIVITY	TIME/REPS	DONE

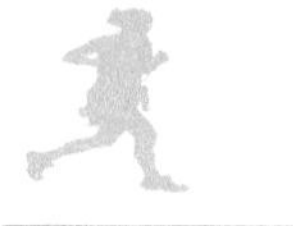 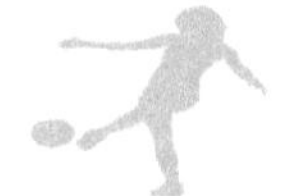 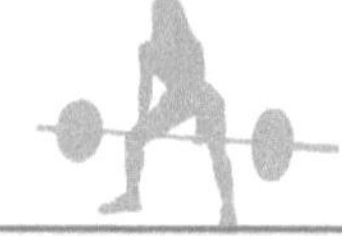 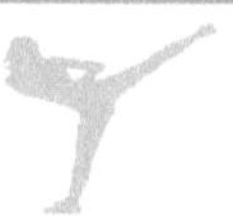 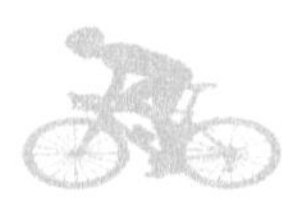

Cardio

ACTIVITY	DISTANCE	TIME	DONE

Weight Training

EXERCISE	SET ONE WEIGHT/REPS	SET TWO WEIGHT/REPS	SET THREE WEIGHT/REPS

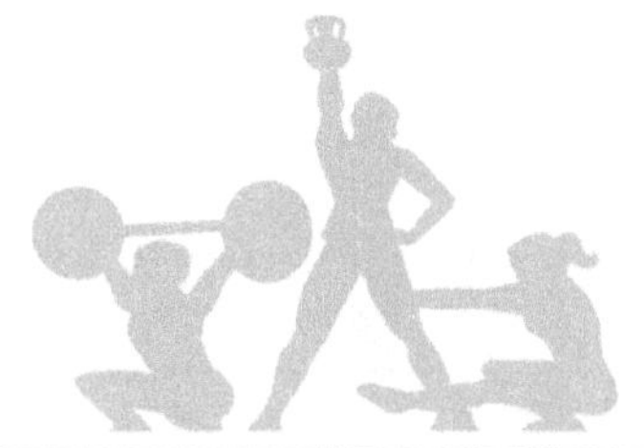

Name: ……………………………

Date: ……………………………

Time: ……………………………

Warm-Up

ACTIVITY	TIME/REPS	DONE

 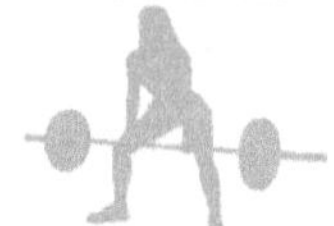 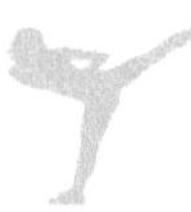 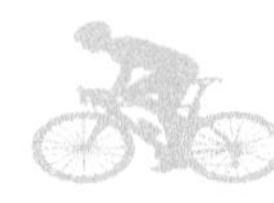

Cardio

ACTIVITY	DISTANCE	TIME	DONE

Weight Training

EXERCISE	SET ONE WEIGHT/REPS	SET TWO WEIGHT/REPS	SET THREE WEIGHT/REPS

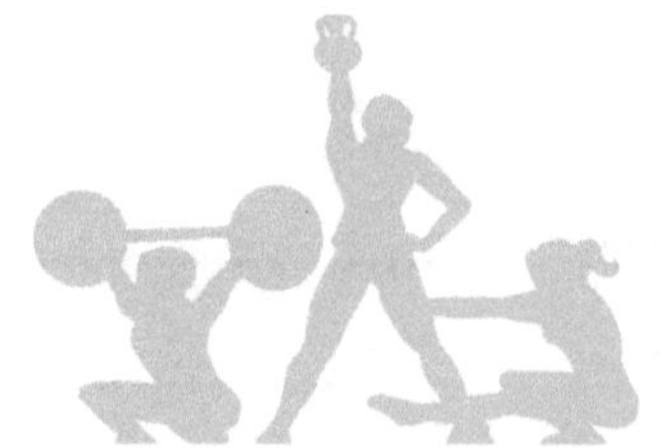

Name: ……………………

Date: ……………………

Time: ……………………

Warm-Up

ACTIVITY	TIME/REPS	DONE

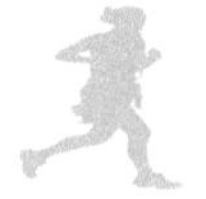 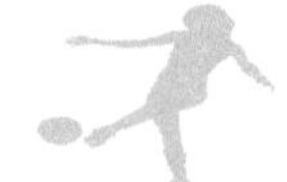 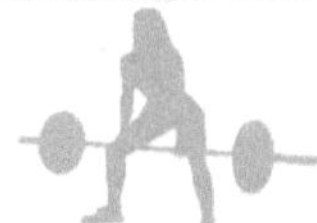 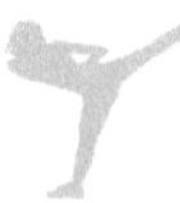 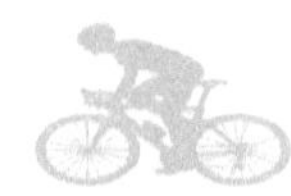

Cardio

ACTIVITY	DISTANCE	TIME	DONE

Weight Training

EXERCISE	SET ONE WEIGHT/REPS	SET TWO WEIGHT/REPS	SET THREE WEIGHT/REPS

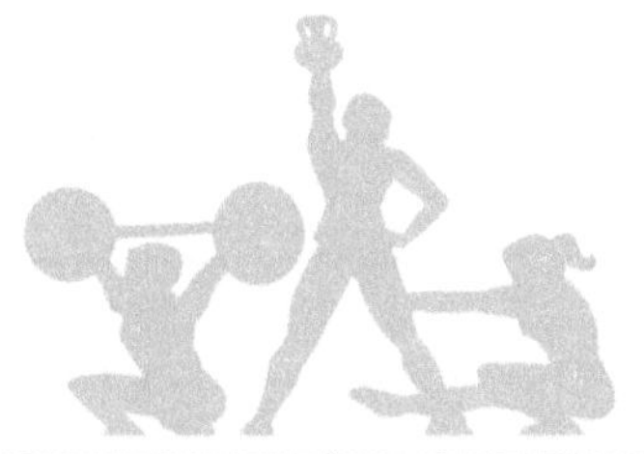

Name: ....

Date: ....

Time: ....

Warm-Up

ACTIVITY	TIME/REPS	DONE

 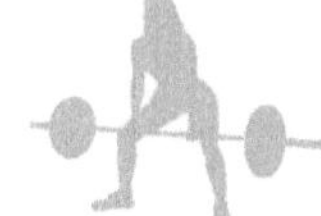 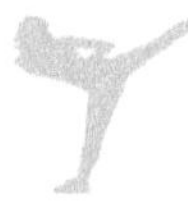 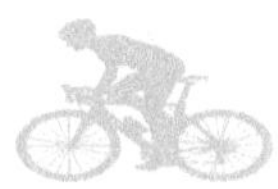

Cardio

ACTIVITY	DISTANCE	TIME	DONE

Weight Training

EXERCISE	SET ONE WEIGHT/REPS	SET TWO WEIGHT/REPS	SET THREE WEIGHT/REPS

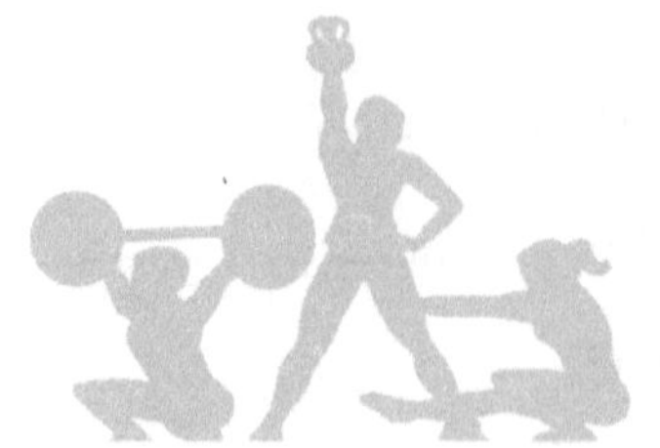

Name: ....

Date: ....

Time: ....

Warm-Up

ACTIVITY	TIME/REPS	DONE

 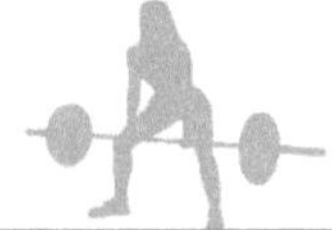 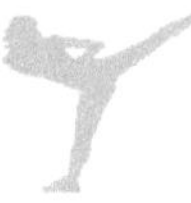 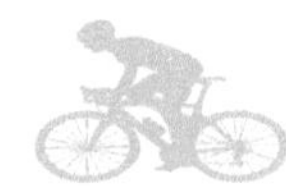

Cardio

ACTIVITY	DISTANCE	TIME	DONE

Weight Training

EXERCISE	SET ONE WEIGHT/REPS	SET TWO WEIGHT/REPS	SET THREE WEIGHT/REPS

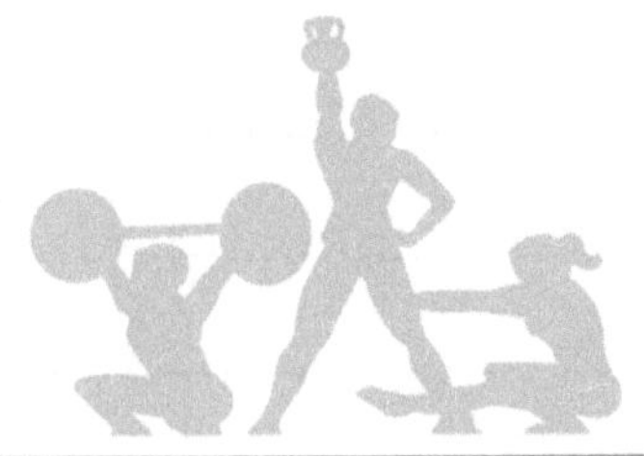

Name: ....

Date: ....

Time: ....

Warm-Up

ACTIVITY	TIME/REPS	DONE

 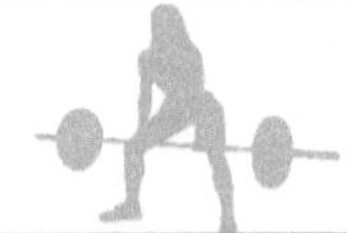 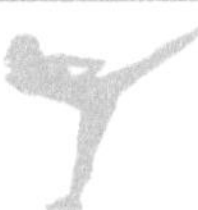 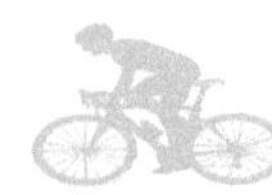

Cardio

ACTIVITY	DISTANCE	TIME	DONE

Weight Training

EXERCISE	SET ONE WEIGHT/REPS	SET TWO WEIGHT/REPS	SET THREE WEIGHT/REPS

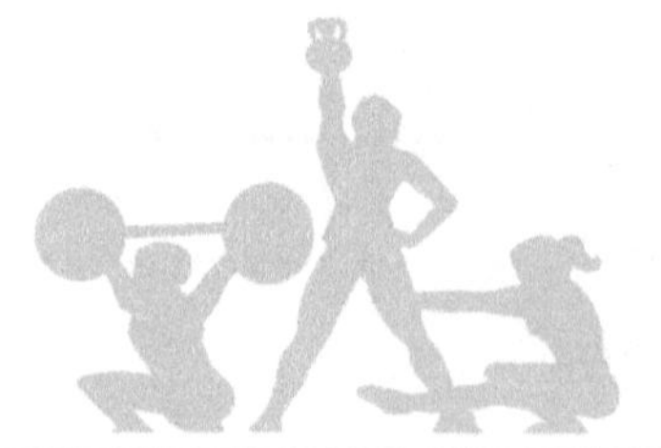

Name: ....

Date: ....

Time: ....

Warm-Up

ACTIVITY	TIME/REPS	DONE

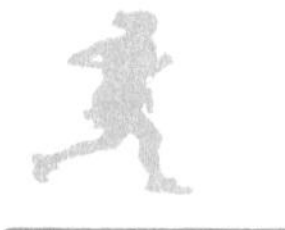 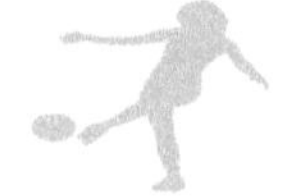 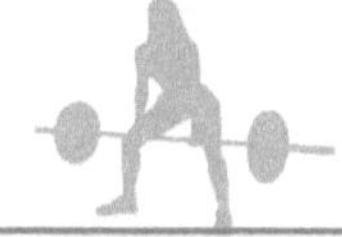 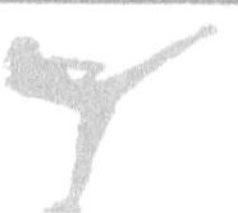 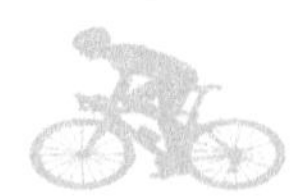

Cardio

ACTIVITY	DISTANCE	TIME	DONE

Weight Training

EXERCISE	SET ONE WEIGHT/REPS	SET TWO WEIGHT/REPS	SET THREE WEIGHT/REPS

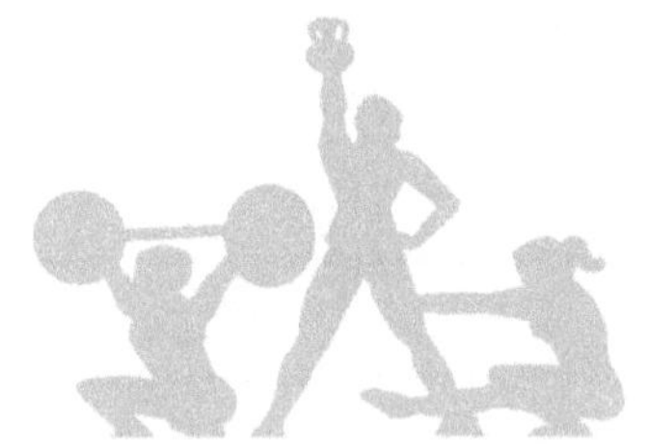

Name: ……………………………

Date: ……………………………

Time: ……………………………

Warm-Up

ACTIVITY	TIME/REPS	DONE

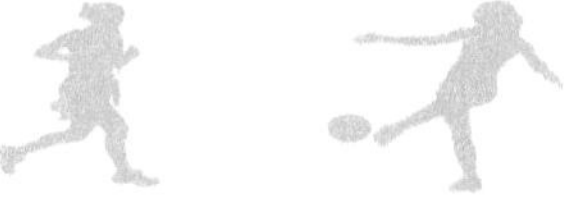 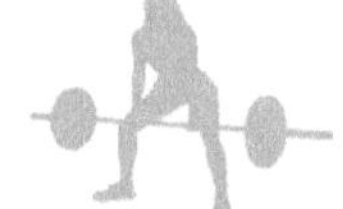 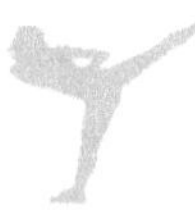 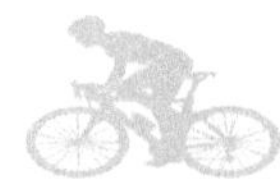

Cardio

ACTIVITY	DISTANCE	TIME	DONE

Weight Training

EXERCISE	SET ONE WEIGHT/REPS	SET TWO WEIGHT/REPS	SET THREE WEIGHT/REPS

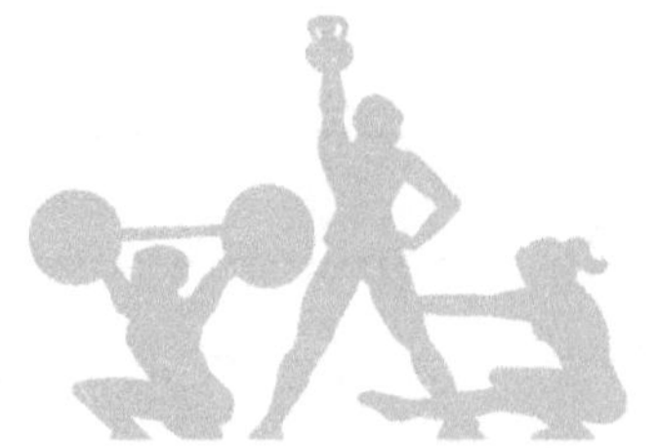

Warm-Up

ACTIVITY	TIME/REPS	DONE

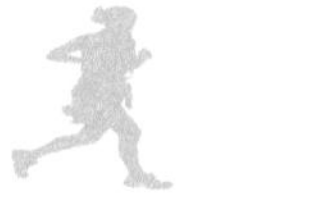 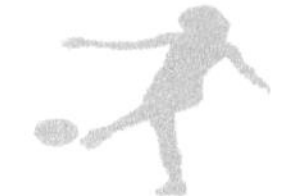 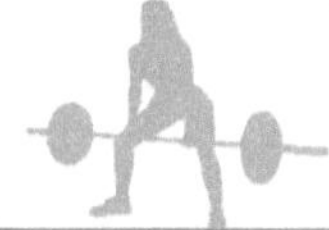 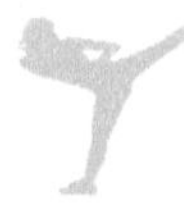 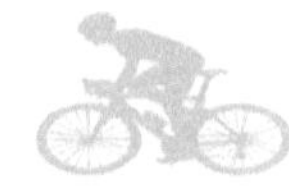

Cardio

ACTIVITY	DISTANCE	TIME	DONE

Weight Training

EXERCISE	SET ONE WEIGHT/REPS	SET TWO WEIGHT/REPS	SET THREE WEIGHT/REPS

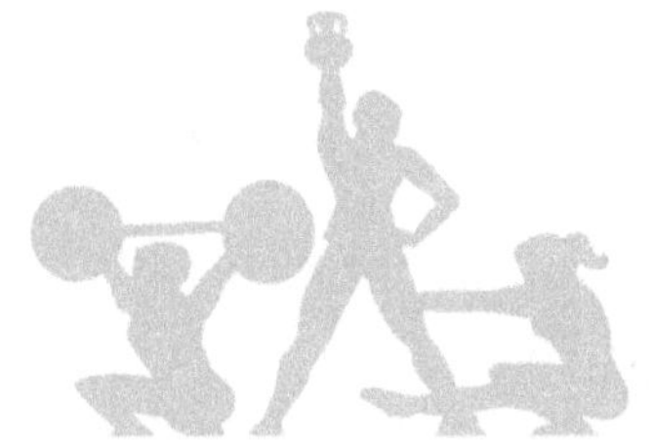

Name: ....

Date: ....

Time: ....

Warm-Up

ACTIVITY	TIME/REPS	DONE

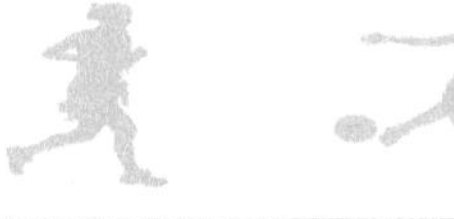 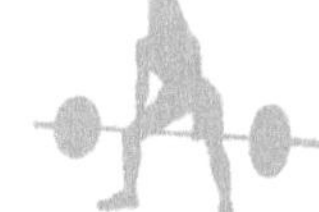 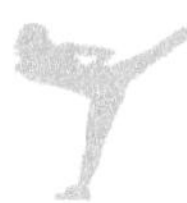 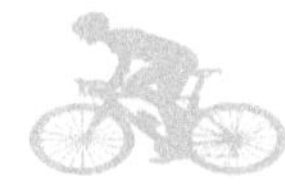

Cardio

ACTIVITY	DISTANCE	TIME	DONE

Weight Training

EXERCISE	SET ONE WEIGHT/REPS	SET TWO WEIGHT/REPS	SET THREE WEIGHT/REPS

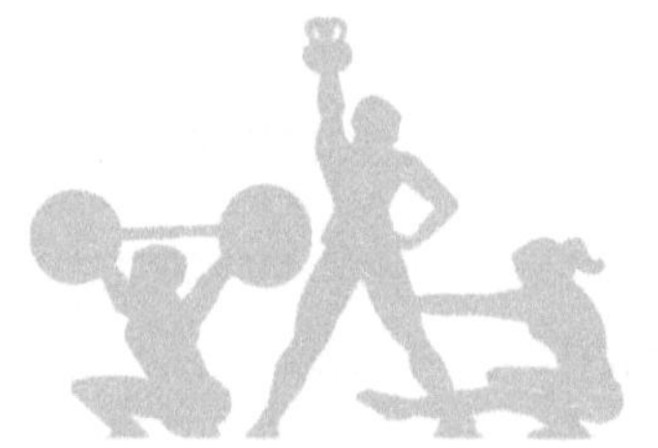

Name: ....

Date: ....

Time: ....

Warm-Up

ACTIVITY	TIME/REPS	DONE

 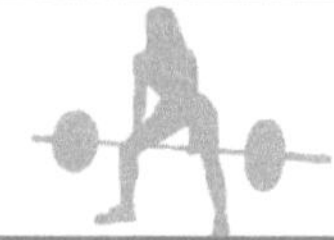 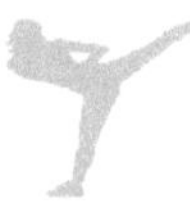 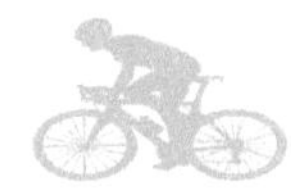

Cardio

ACTIVITY	DISTANCE	TIME	DONE

Weight Training

EXERCISE	SET ONE WEIGHT/REPS	SET TWO WEIGHT/REPS	SET THREE WEIGHT/REPS

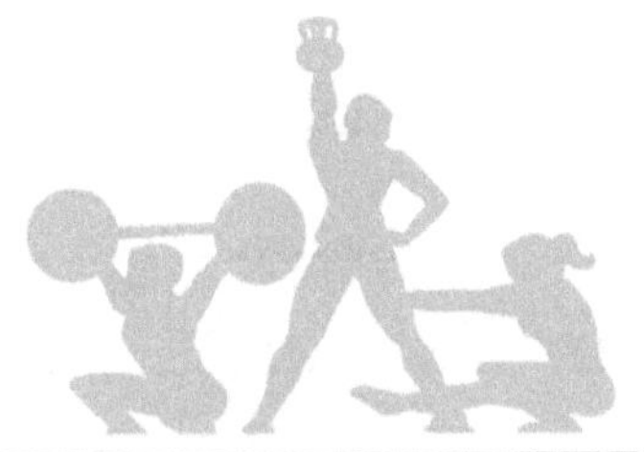

Name: ....

Date: ....

Time: ....

Warm-Up

ACTIVITY	TIME/REPS	DONE

 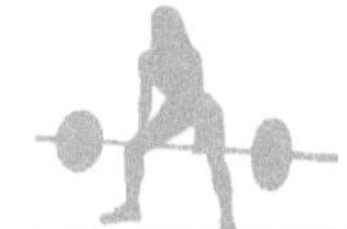 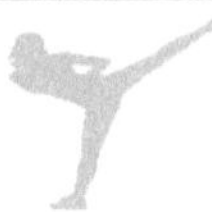 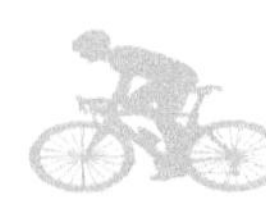

Cardio

ACTIVITY	DISTANCE	TIME	DONE

Weight Training

EXERCISE	SET ONE WEIGHT/REPS	SET TWO WEIGHT/REPS	SET THREE WEIGHT/REPS

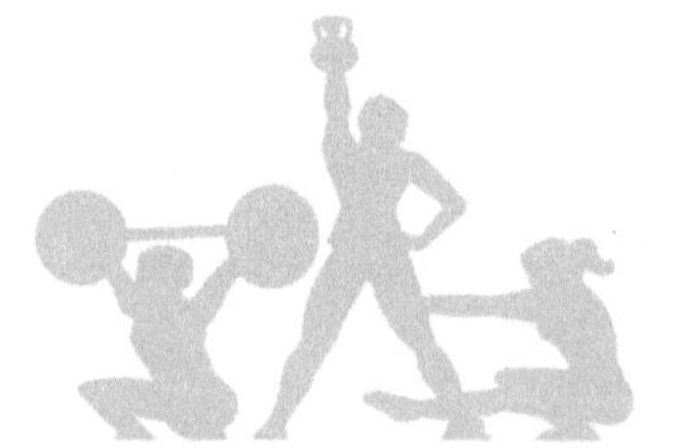

Name: ....

Date: ....

Time: ....

Warm-Up

ACTIVITY	TIME/REPS	DONE

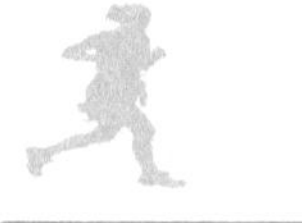 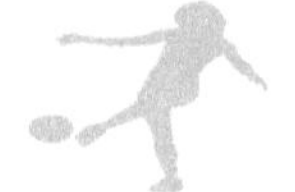 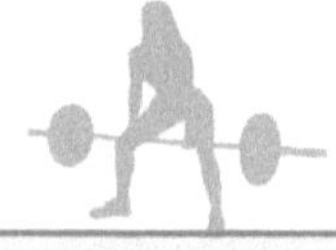 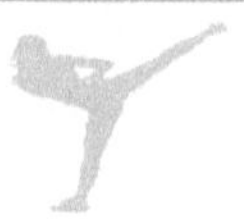 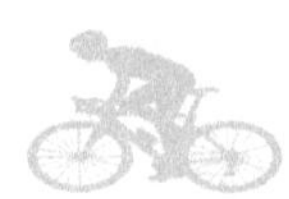

Cardio

ACTIVITY	DISTANCE	TIME	DONE

Weight Training

EXERCISE	SET ONE WEIGHT/REPS	SET TWO WEIGHT/REPS	SET THREE WEIGHT/REPS

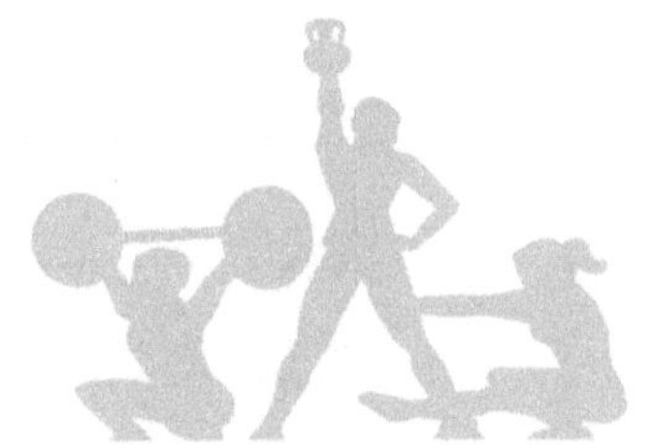

Warm-Up

ACTIVITY	TIME/REPS	DONE

 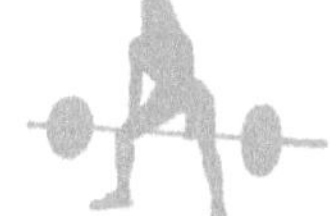 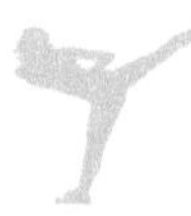 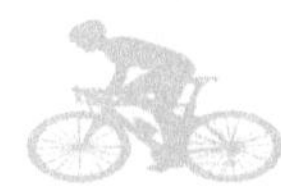

Cardio

ACTIVITY	DISTANCE	TIME	DONE

Weight Training

EXERCISE	SET ONE WEIGHT/REPS	SET TWO WEIGHT/REPS	SET THREE WEIGHT/REPS

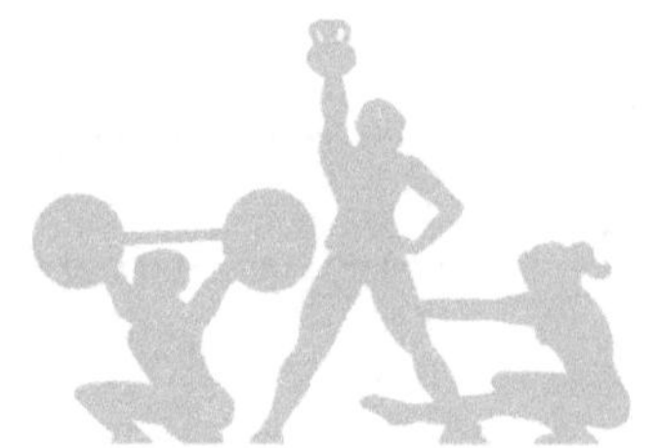

Name: ....

Date: ....

Time: ....

Warm-Up

ACTIVITY	TIME/REPS	DONE

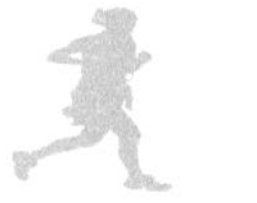  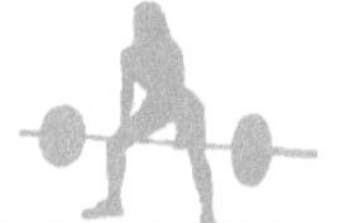 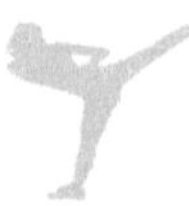 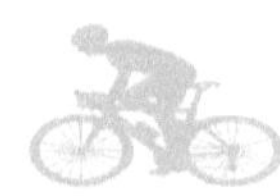

Cardio

ACTIVITY	DISTANCE	TIME	DONE

Weight Training

EXERCISE	SET ONE WEIGHT/REPS	SET TWO WEIGHT/REPS	SET THREE WEIGHT/REPS

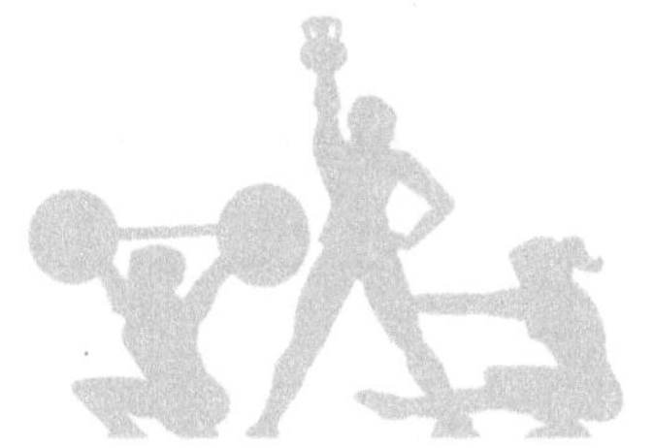

Name: ....

Date: ....

Time: ....

Warm-Up

ACTIVITY	TIME/REPS	DONE

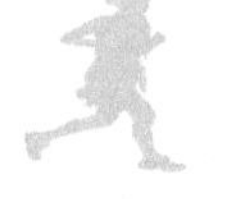 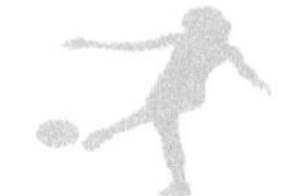 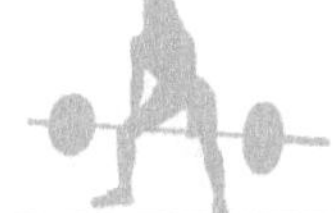 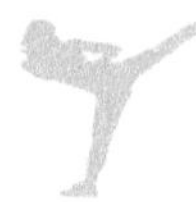 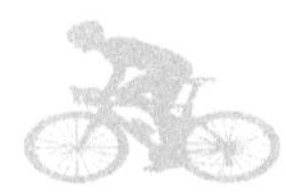

Cardio

ACTIVITY	DISTANCE	TIME	DONE

Weight Training

EXERCISE	SET ONE WEIGHT/REPS	SET TWO WEIGHT/REPS	SET THREE WEIGHT/REPS

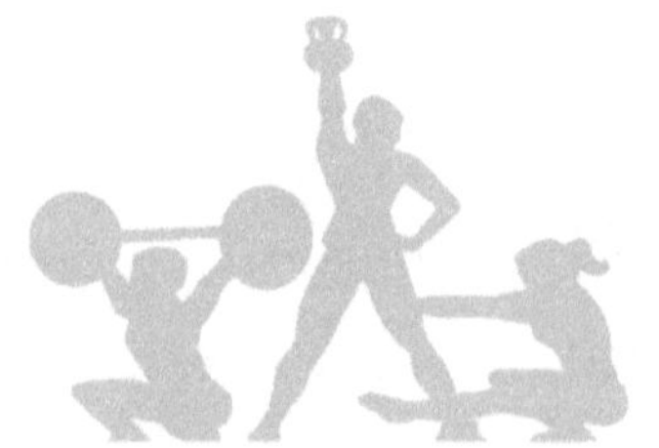

Name: ....

Date: ....

Time: ....

Warm-Up

ACTIVITY	TIME/REPS	DONE

 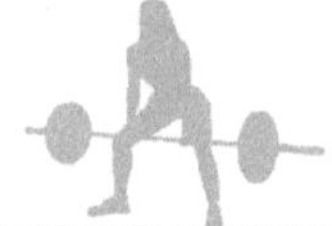 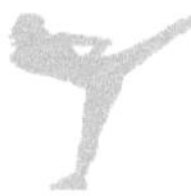 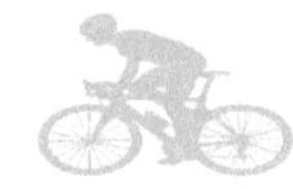

Cardio

ACTIVITY	DISTANCE	TIME	DONE

Weight Training

EXERCISE	SET ONE WEIGHT/REPS	SET TWO WEIGHT/REPS	SET THREE WEIGHT/REPS

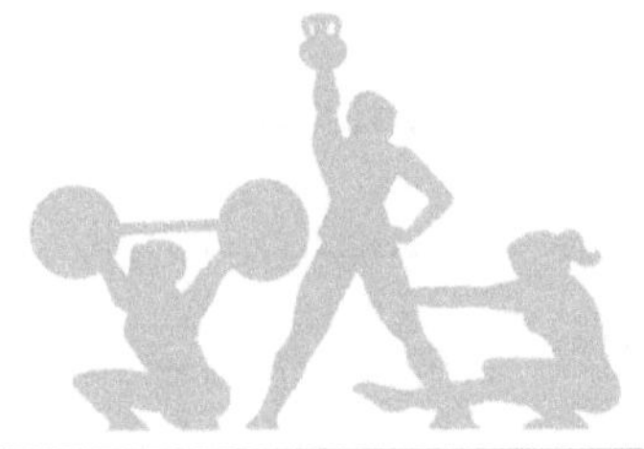

Name: ....

Date: ....

Time: ....

Warm-Up

ACTIVITY	TIME/REPS	DONE

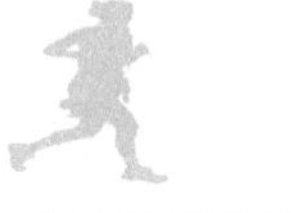 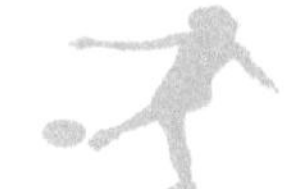 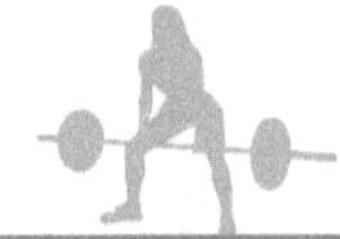 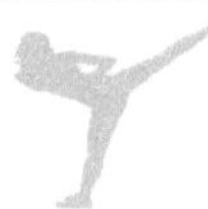 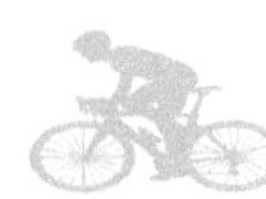

Cardio

ACTIVITY	DISTANCE	TIME	DONE

Weight Training

EXERCISE	SET ONE WEIGHT/REPS	SET TWO WEIGHT/REPS	SET THREE WEIGHT/REPS

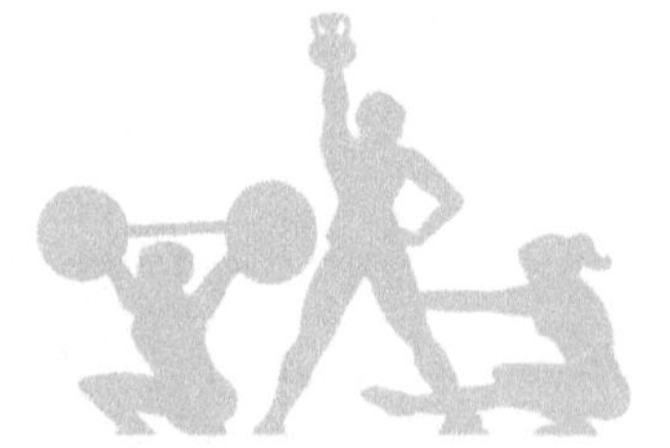

Name: ....

Date: ....

Time: ....

Warm-Up

ACTIVITY	TIME/REPS	DONE

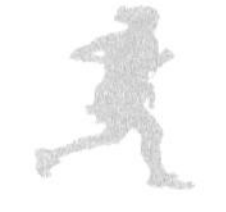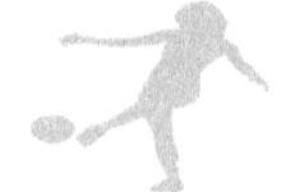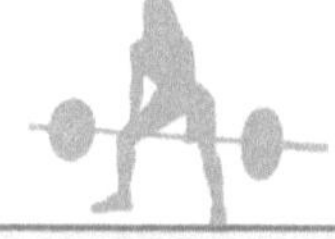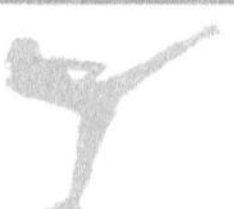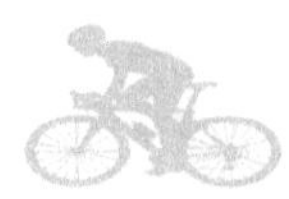

Cardio

ACTIVITY	DISTANCE	TIME	DONE

Weight Training

EXERCISE	SET ONE WEIGHT/REPS	SET TWO WEIGHT/REPS	SET THREE WEIGHT/REPS

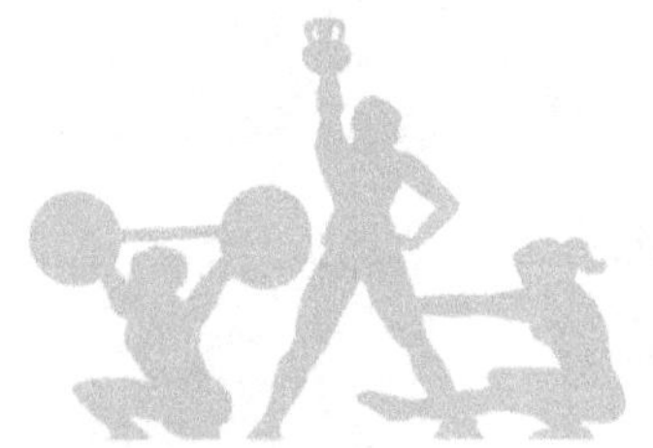

Name: ....

Date: ....

Time: ....

Warm-Up

ACTIVITY	TIME/REPS	DONE

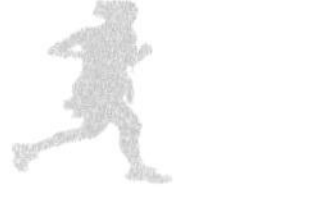  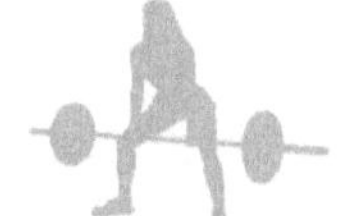 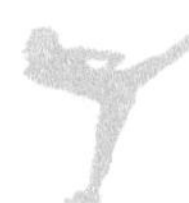 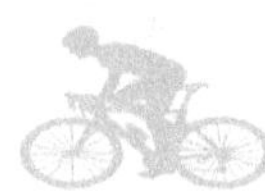

Cardio

ACTIVITY	DISTANCE	TIME	DONE

Weight Training

EXERCISE	SET ONE WEIGHT/REPS	SET TWO WEIGHT/REPS	SET THREE WEIGHT/REPS

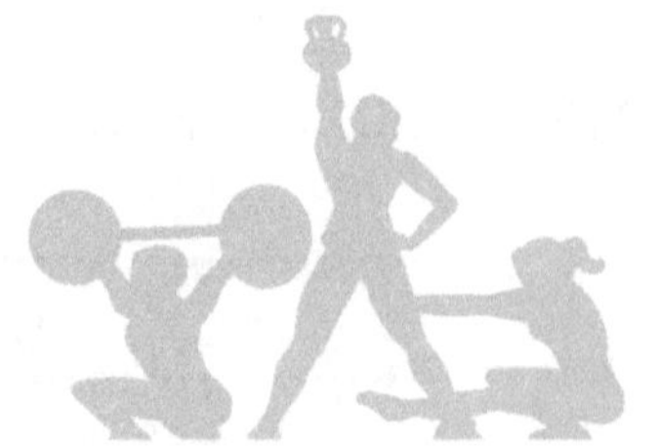

Name: ....

Date: ....

Time: ....

Warm-Up

ACTIVITY	TIME/REPS	DONE

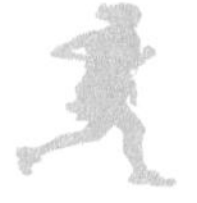 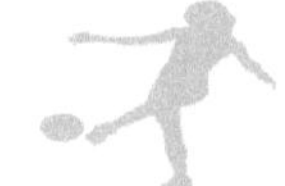 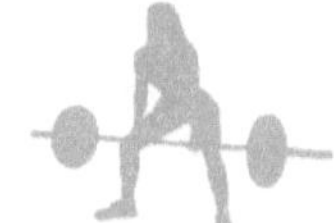 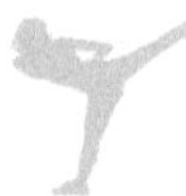 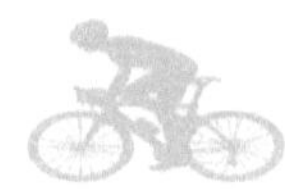

Cardio

ACTIVITY	DISTANCE	TIME	DONE

Weight Training

EXERCISE	SET ONE WEIGHT/REPS	SET TWO WEIGHT/REPS	SET THREE WEIGHT/REPS

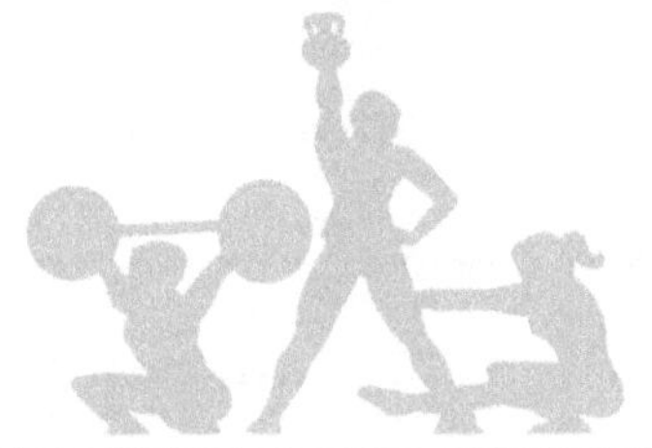

Name: ....

Date: ....

Time: ....

Warm-Up

ACTIVITY	TIME/REPS	DONE

 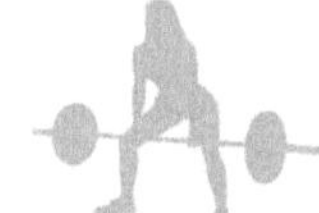 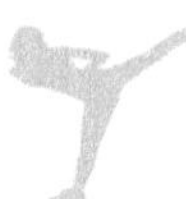 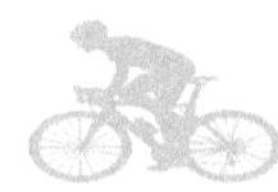

Cardio

ACTIVITY	DISTANCE	TIME	DONE

Weight Training

EXERCISE	SET ONE WEIGHT/REPS	SET TWO WEIGHT/REPS	SET THREE WEIGHT/REPS

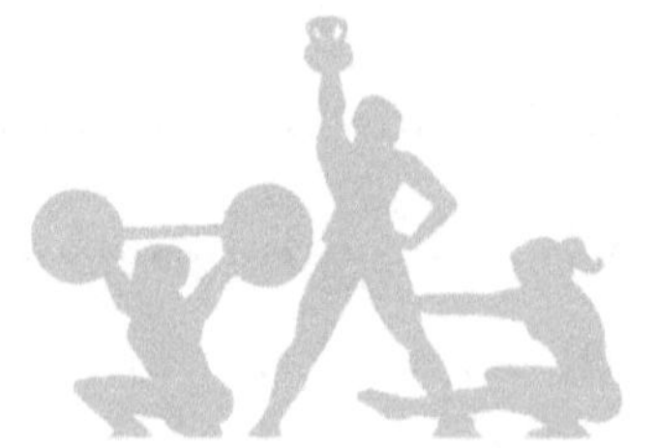

Name: ....

Date: ....

Time: ....

Warm-Up

ACTIVITY	TIME/REPS	DONE

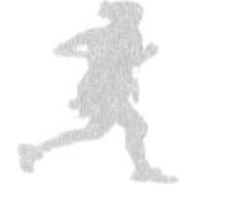  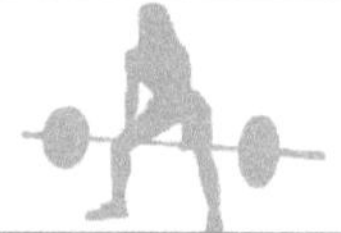 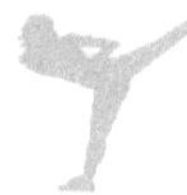 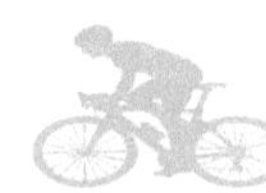

Cardio

ACTIVITY	DISTANCE	TIME	DONE

Weight Training

EXERCISE	SET ONE WEIGHT/REPS	SET TWO WEIGHT/REPS	SET THREE WEIGHT/REPS

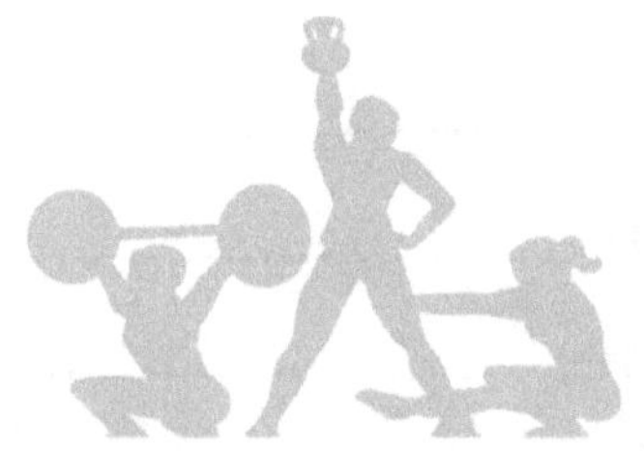

Name: ....

Date: ....

Time: ....

Warm-Up

ACTIVITY	TIME/REPS	DONE

 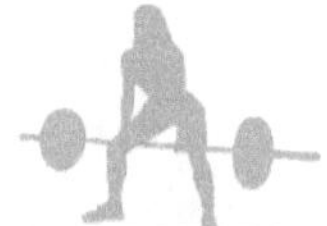 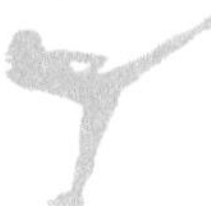 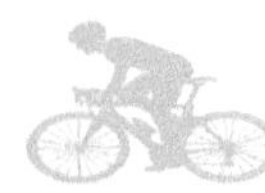

Cardio

ACTIVITY	DISTANCE	TIME	DONE

Weight Training

EXERCISE	SET ONE WEIGHT/REPS	SET TWO WEIGHT/REPS	SET THREE WEIGHT/REPS

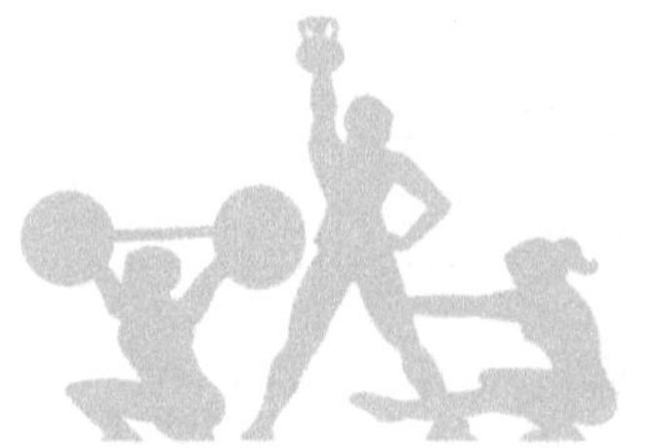

Name: ....

Date: ....

Time: ....

Warm-Up

ACTIVITY	TIME/REPS	DONE

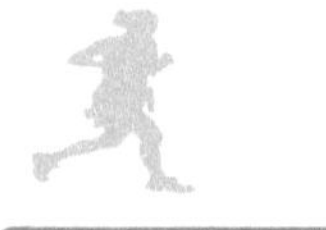 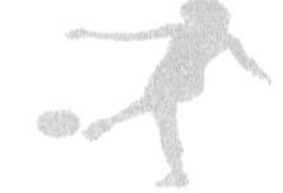 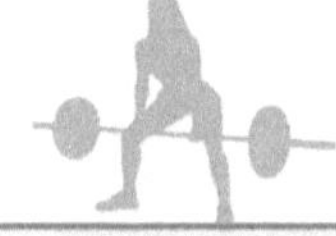 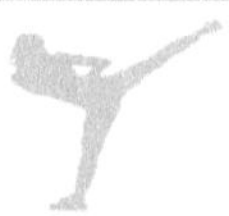 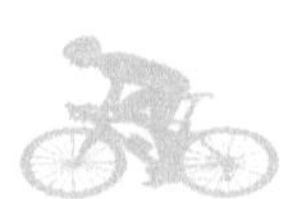

Cardio

ACTIVITY	DISTANCE	TIME	DONE

Weight Training

EXERCISE	SET ONE WEIGHT/REPS	SET TWO WEIGHT/REPS	SET THREE WEIGHT/REPS

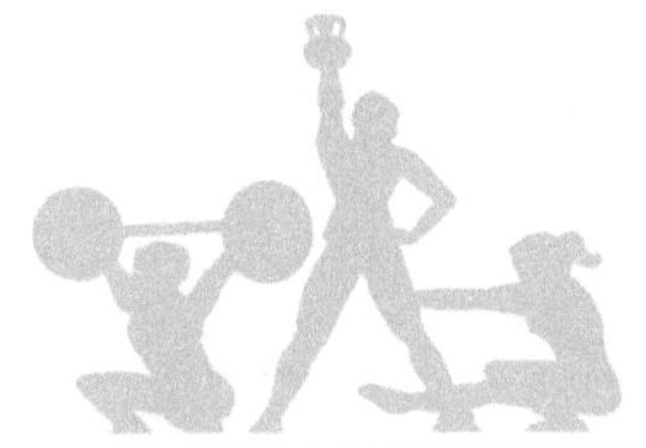

Name: ……………………………

Date: ……………………………

Time: ……………………………

Warm-Up

ACTIVITY	TIME/REPS	DONE

 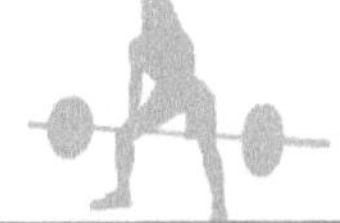 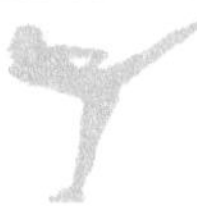 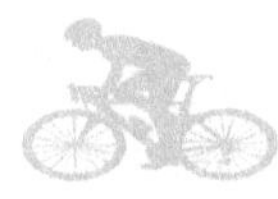

Cardio

ACTIVITY	DISTANCE	TIME	DONE

Weight Training

EXERCISE	SET ONE WEIGHT/REPS	SET TWO WEIGHT/REPS	SET THREE WEIGHT/REPS

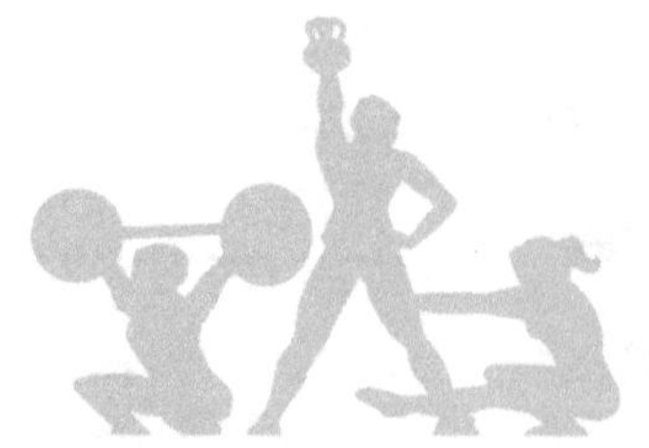

Warm-Up

ACTIVITY	TIME/REPS	DONE

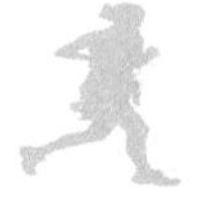 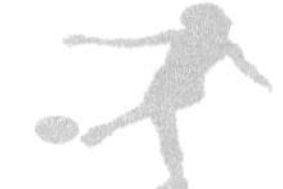 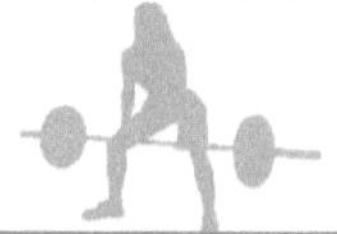 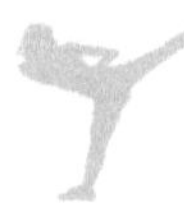 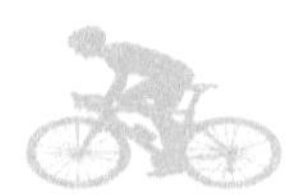

Cardio

ACTIVITY	DISTANCE	TIME	DONE

Weight Training

EXERCISE	SET ONE WEIGHT/REPS	SET TWO WEIGHT/REPS	SET THREE WEIGHT/REPS

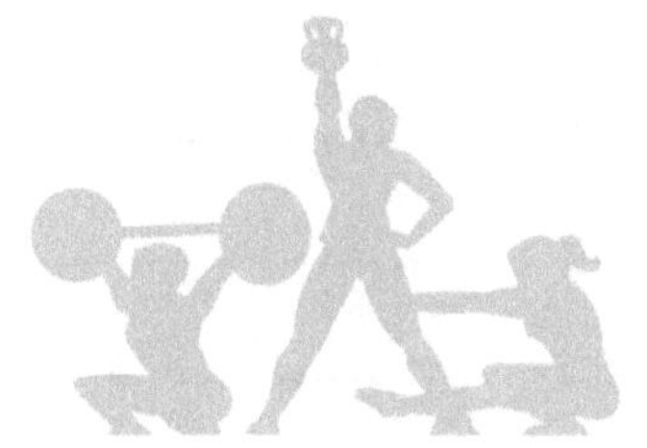

Name: ....

Date: ....

Time: ....

Warm-Up

ACTIVITY	TIME/REPS	DONE

 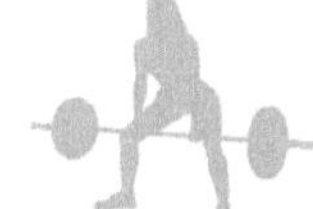 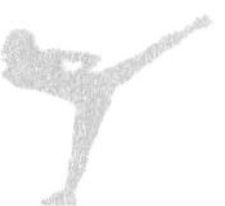 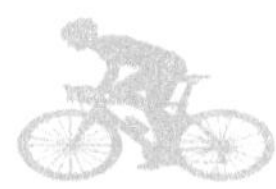

Cardio

ACTIVITY	DISTANCE	TIME	DONE

Weight Training

EXERCISE	SET ONE WEIGHT/REPS	SET TWO WEIGHT/REPS	SET THREE WEIGHT/REPS

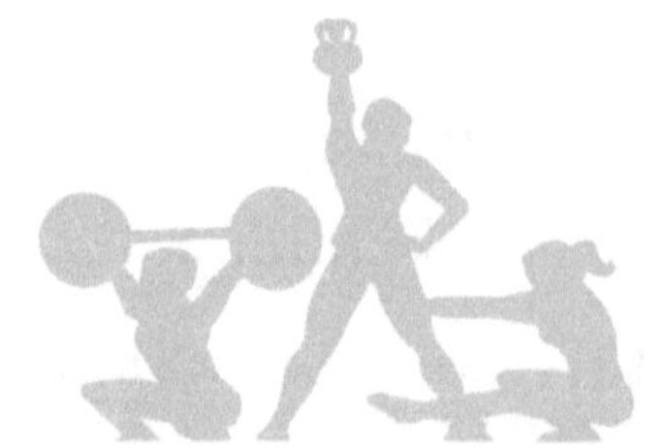

Name: ....

Date: ....

Time: ....

Warm-Up

ACTIVITY	TIME/REPS	DONE

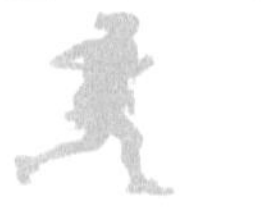  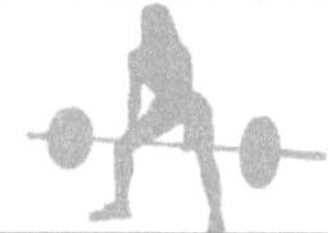 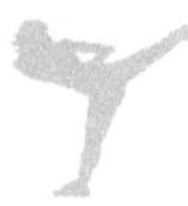 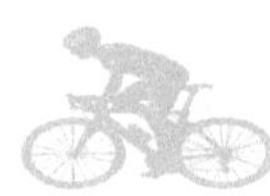

Cardio

ACTIVITY	DISTANCE	TIME	DONE

Weight Training

EXERCISE	SET ONE WEIGHT/REPS	SET TWO WEIGHT/REPS	SET THREE WEIGHT/REPS

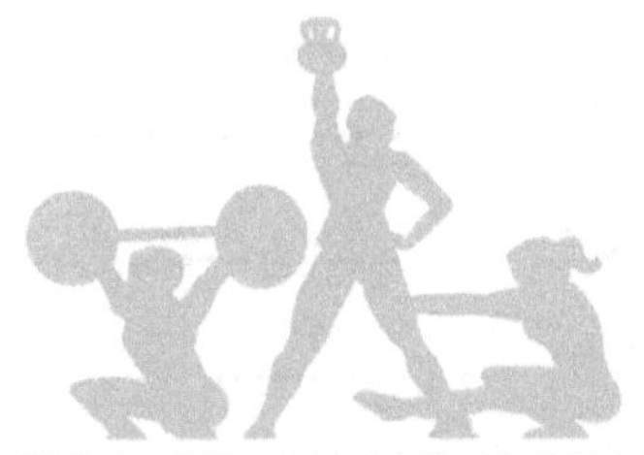

Name: ....

Date: ....

Time: ....

Warm-Up

ACTIVITY	TIME/REPS	DONE

 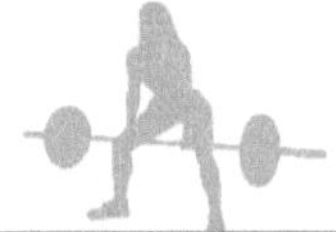 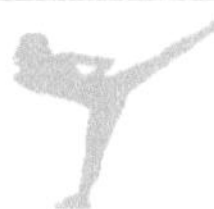 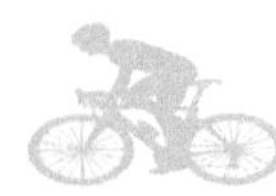

Cardio

ACTIVITY	DISTANCE	TIME	DONE

Weight Training

EXERCISE	SET ONE WEIGHT/REPS	SET TWO WEIGHT/REPS	SET THREE WEIGHT/REPS

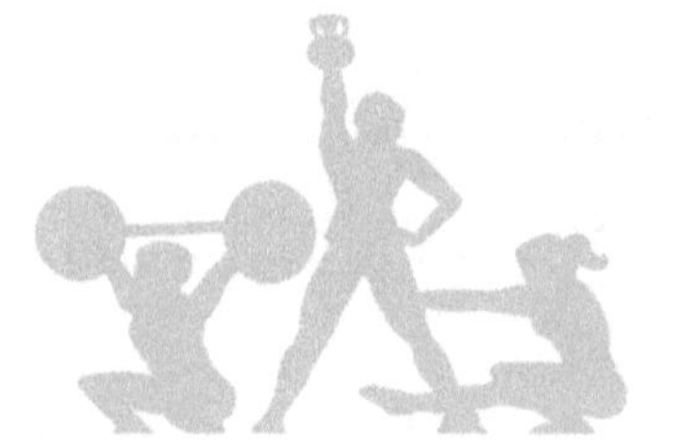

Name: ....

Date: ....

Time: ....

Warm-Up

ACTIVITY	TIME/REPS	DONE

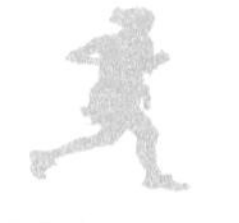 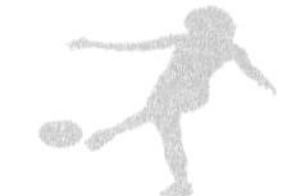 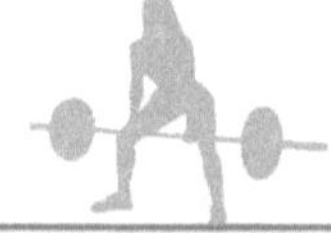 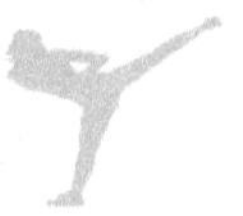 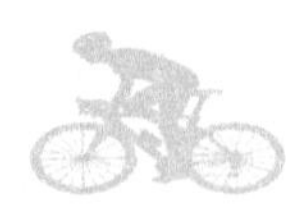

Cardio

ACTIVITY	DISTANCE	TIME	DONE

Weight Training

EXERCISE	SET ONE WEIGHT/REPS	SET TWO WEIGHT/REPS	SET THREE WEIGHT/REPS

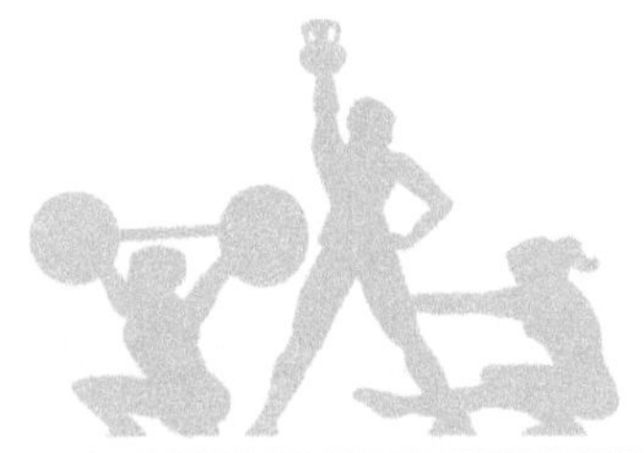

Name: ....

Date: ....

Time: ....

Warm-Up

ACTIVITY	TIME/REPS	DONE

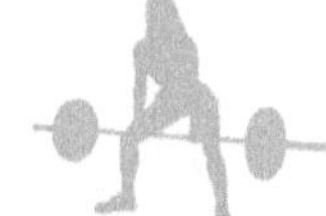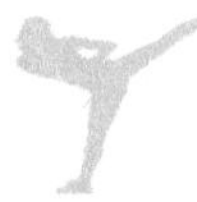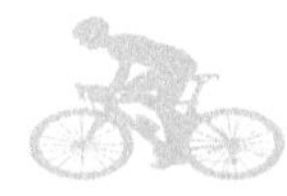

Cardio

ACTIVITY	DISTANCE	TIME	DONE

Weight Training

EXERCISE	SET ONE WEIGHT/REPS	SET TWO WEIGHT/REPS	SET THREE WEIGHT/REPS

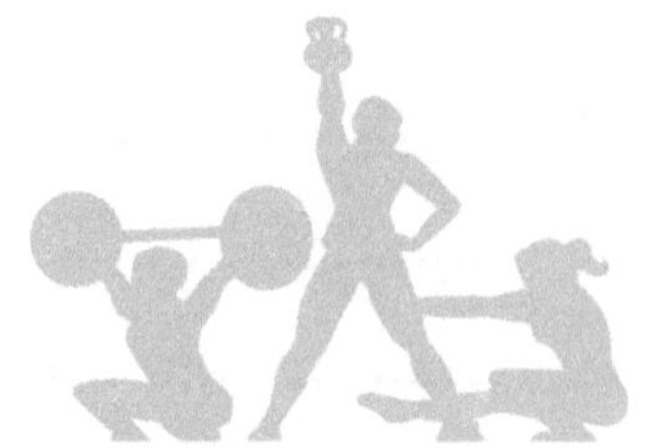

Name: ....

Date: ....

Time: ....

Warm-Up

ACTIVITY	TIME/REPS	DONE

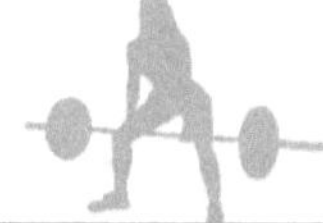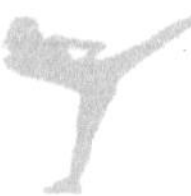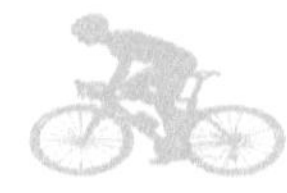

Cardio

ACTIVITY	DISTANCE	TIME	DONE

Weight Training

EXERCISE	SET ONE WEIGHT/REPS	SET TWO WEIGHT/REPS	SET THREE WEIGHT/REPS

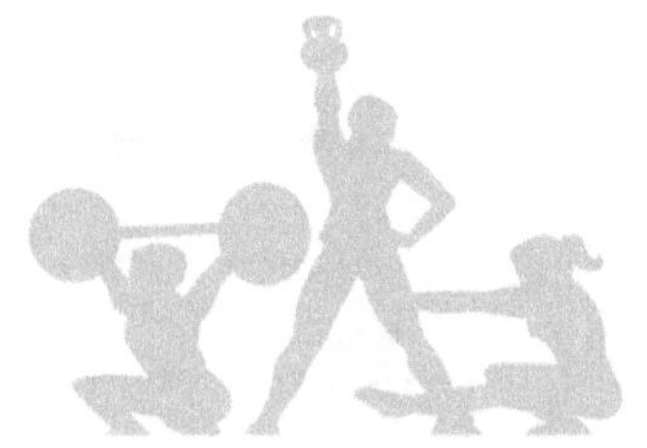

Name: ....

Date: ....

Time: ....

Warm-Up

ACTIVITY	TIME/REPS	DONE

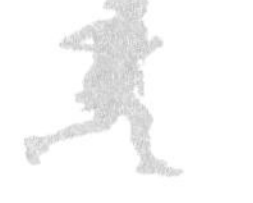 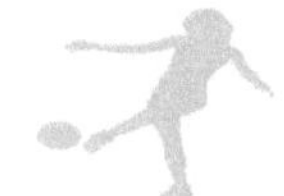 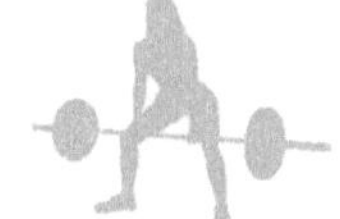 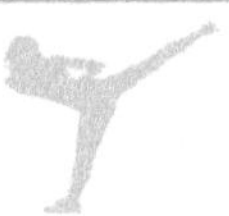 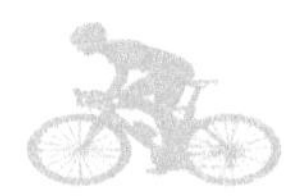

Cardio

ACTIVITY	DISTANCE	TIME	DONE

Weight Training

EXERCISE	SET ONE WEIGHT/REPS	SET TWO WEIGHT/REPS	SET THREE WEIGHT/REPS

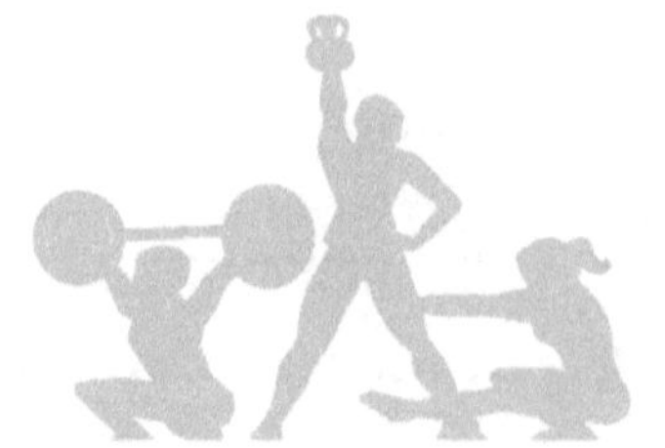

Warm-Up

ACTIVITY	TIME/REPS	DONE

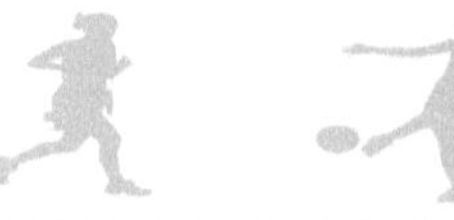 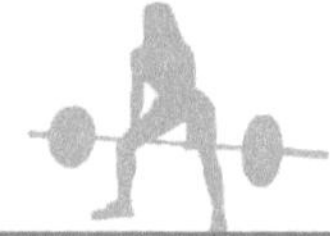 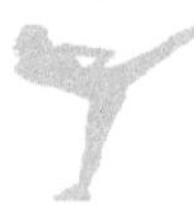 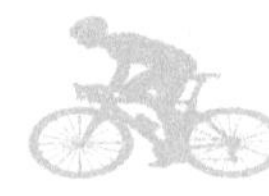

Cardio

ACTIVITY	DISTANCE	TIME	DONE

Weight Training

EXERCISE	SET ONE WEIGHT/REPS	SET TWO WEIGHT/REPS	SET THREE WEIGHT/REPS

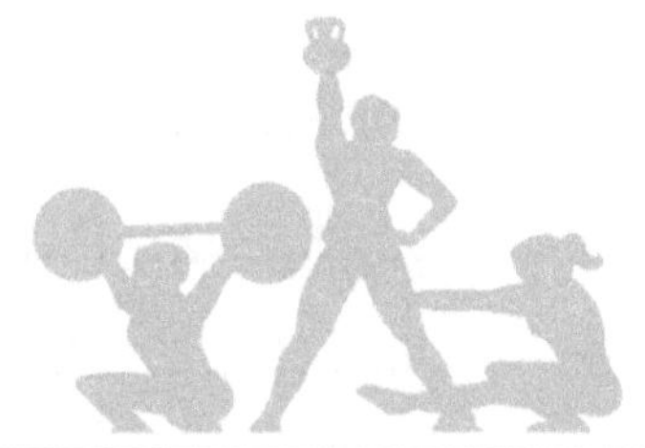

Name: ....

Date: ....

Time: ....

Warm-Up

ACTIVITY	TIME/REPS	DONE

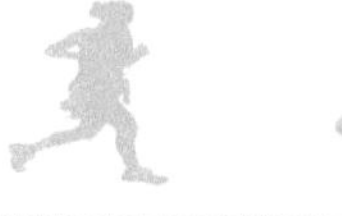 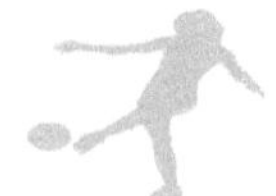 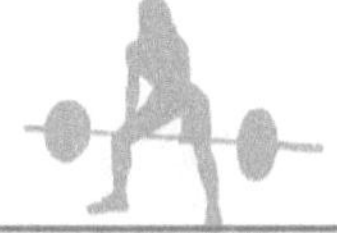 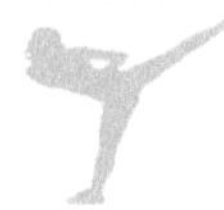 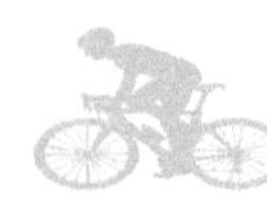

Cardio

ACTIVITY	DISTANCE	TIME	DONE

Weight Training

EXERCISE	SET ONE WEIGHT/REPS	SET TWO WEIGHT/REPS	SET THREE WEIGHT/REPS

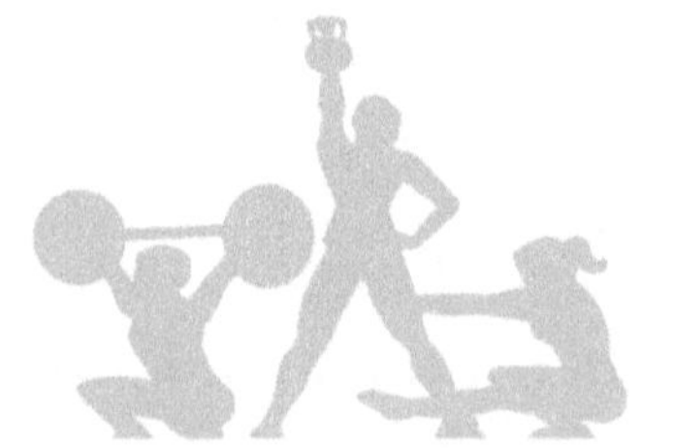

Name: ....

Date: ....

Time: ....

Warm-Up

ACTIVITY	TIME/REPS	DONE

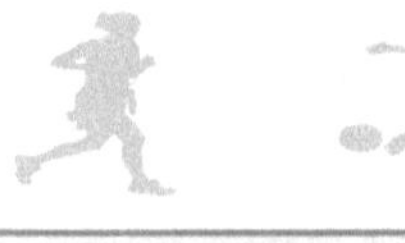 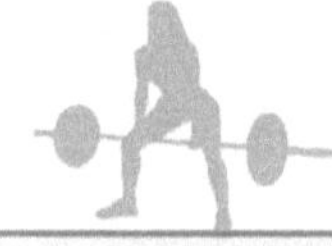 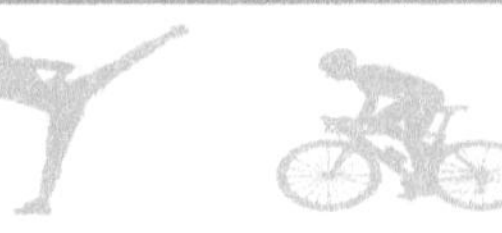

Cardio

ACTIVITY	DISTANCE	TIME	DONE

Weight Training

EXERCISE	SET ONE WEIGHT/REPS	SET TWO WEIGHT/REPS	SET THREE WEIGHT/REPS

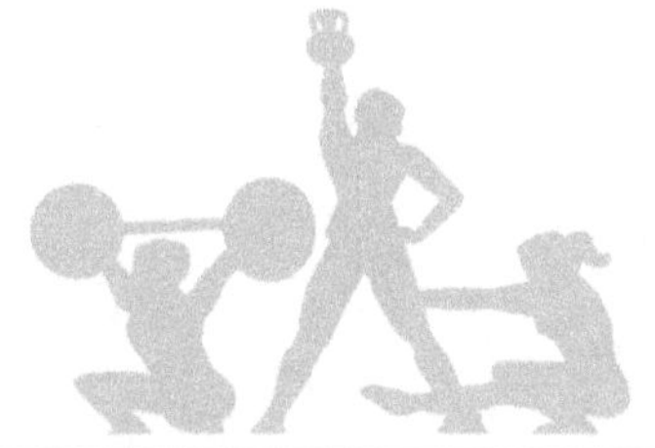

Warm-Up

ACTIVITY	TIME/REPS	DONE

 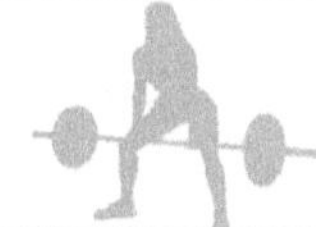 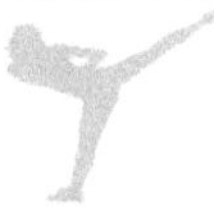 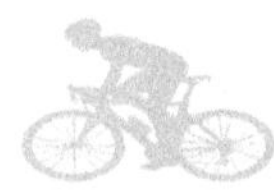

Cardio

ACTIVITY	DISTANCE	TIME	DONE

Weight Training

EXERCISE	SET ONE WEIGHT/REPS	SET TWO WEIGHT/REPS	SET THREE WEIGHT/REPS

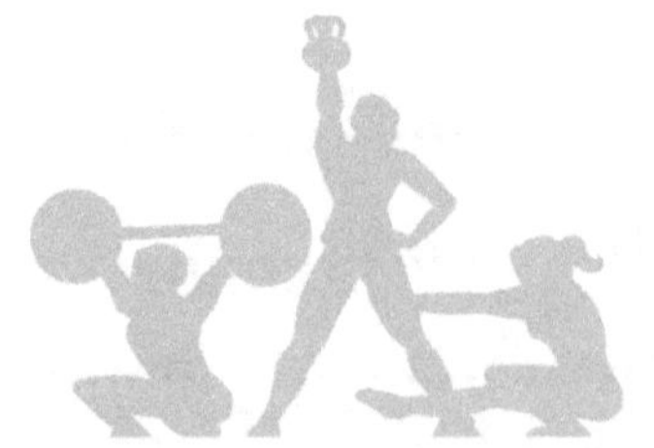

Warm-Up

ACTIVITY	TIME/REPS	DONE

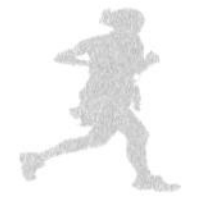 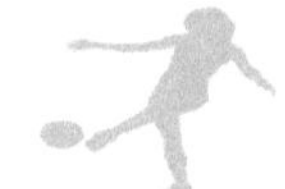 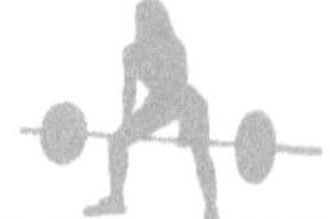 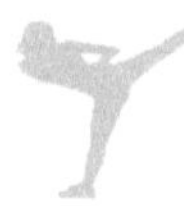 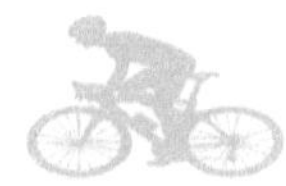

Cardio

ACTIVITY	DISTANCE	TIME	DONE

Weight Training

EXERCISE	SET ONE WEIGHT/REPS	SET TWO WEIGHT/REPS	SET THREE WEIGHT/REPS

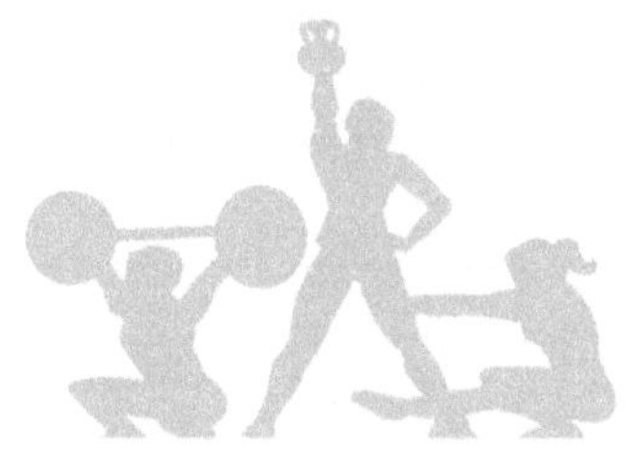

Name: ....

Date: ....

Time: ....

Warm-Up

ACTIVITY	TIME/REPS	DONE

 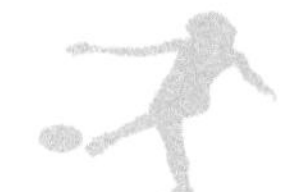 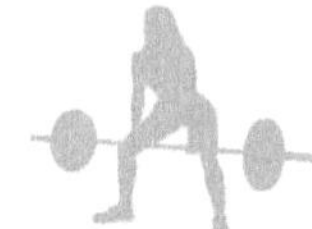 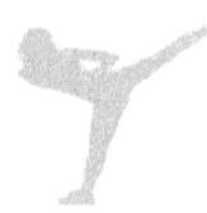 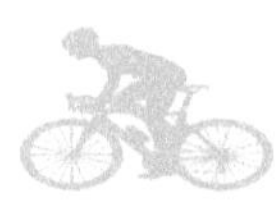

Cardio

ACTIVITY	DISTANCE	TIME	DONE

Weight Training

EXERCISE	SET ONE WEIGHT/REPS	SET TWO WEIGHT/REPS	SET THREE WEIGHT/REPS

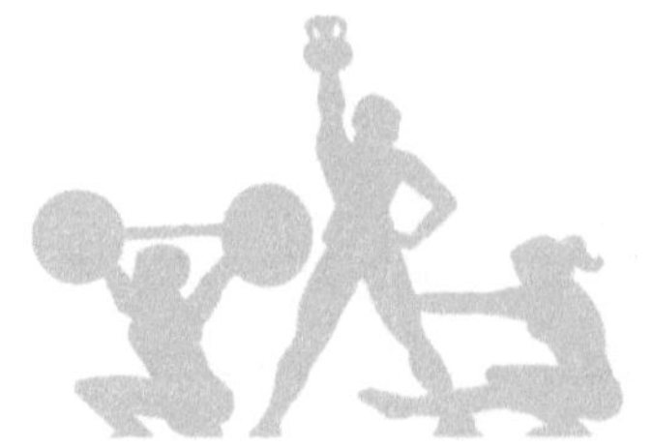

Name: ....

Date: ....

Time: ....

Warm-Up

ACTIVITY	TIME/REPS	DONE

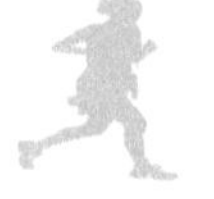 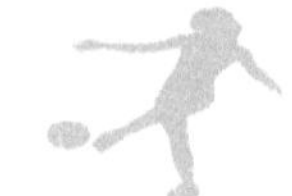 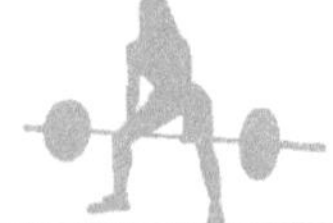 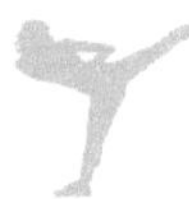 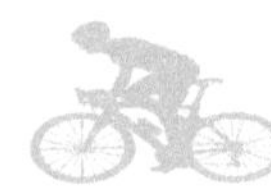

Cardio

ACTIVITY	DISTANCE	TIME	DONE

Weight Training

EXERCISE	SET ONE WEIGHT/REPS	SET TWO WEIGHT/REPS	SET THREE WEIGHT/REPS

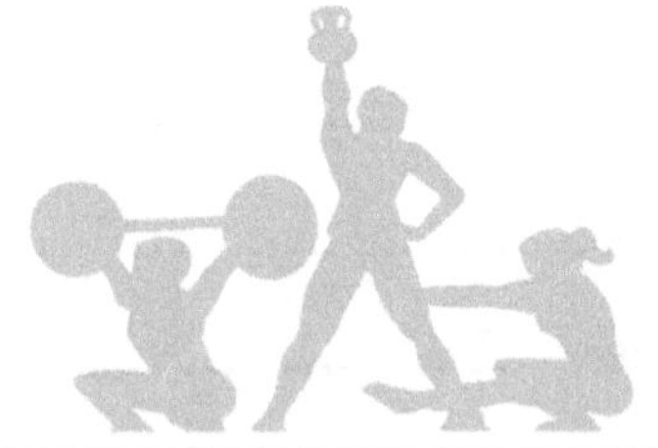

Name: ....

Date: ....

Time: ....

Warm-Up

ACTIVITY	TIME/REPS	DONE

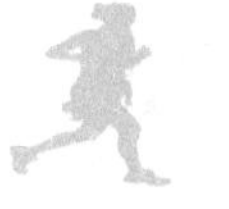 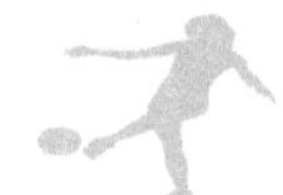 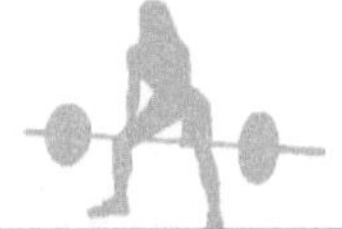 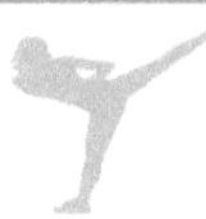 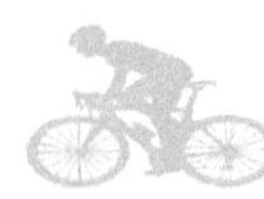

Cardio

ACTIVITY	DISTANCE	TIME	DONE

Weight Training

EXERCISE	SET ONE WEIGHT/REPS	SET TWO WEIGHT/REPS	SET THREE WEIGHT/REPS

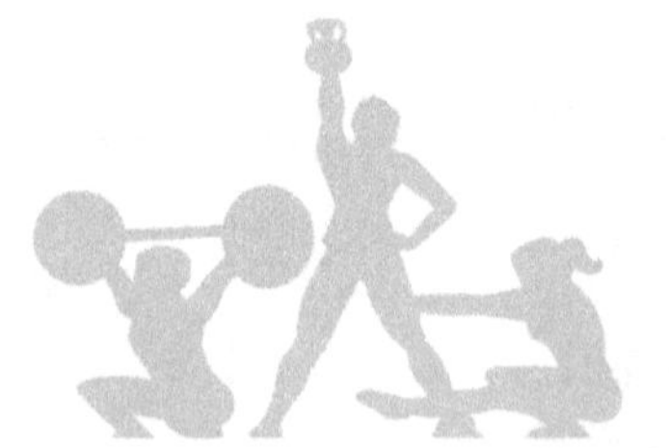

Name: ……………………………

Date: ……………………………

Time: ……………………………

Warm-Up

ACTIVITY	TIME/REPS	DONE

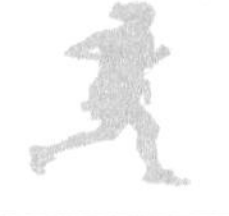  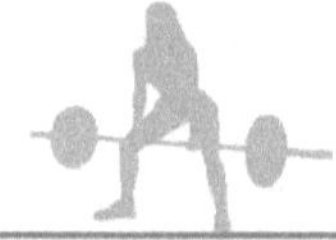 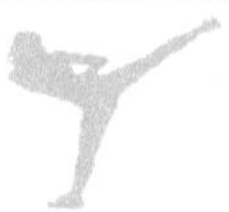 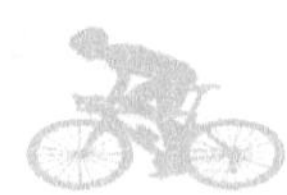

Cardio

ACTIVITY	DISTANCE	TIME	DONE

Weight Training

EXERCISE	SET ONE WEIGHT/REPS	SET TWO WEIGHT/REPS	SET THREE WEIGHT/REPS

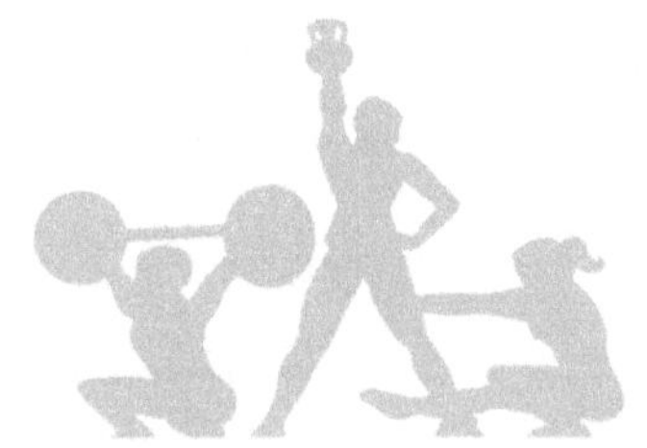

Name: ....

Date: ....

Time: ....

Warm-Up

ACTIVITY	TIME/REPS	DONE

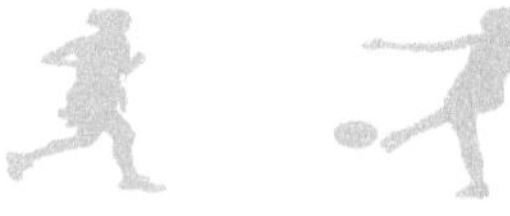  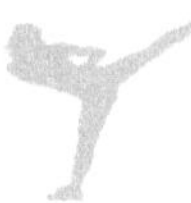 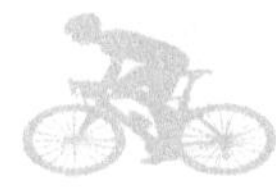

Cardio

ACTIVITY	DISTANCE	TIME	DONE

Weight Training

EXERCISE	SET ONE WEIGHT/REPS	SET TWO WEIGHT/REPS	SET THREE WEIGHT/REPS

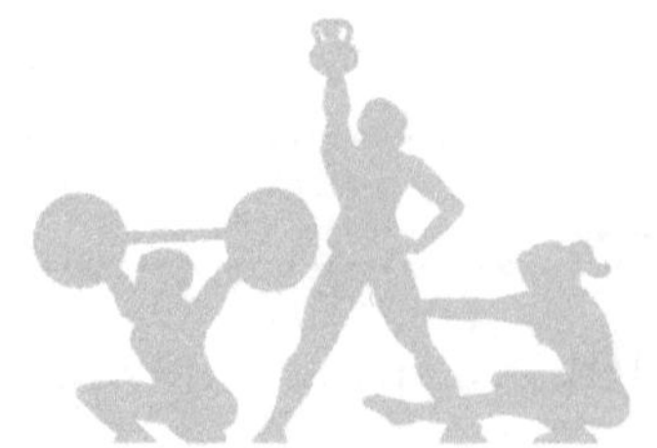

Name: ....

Date: ....

Time: ....

Warm-Up

ACTIVITY	TIME/REPS	DONE

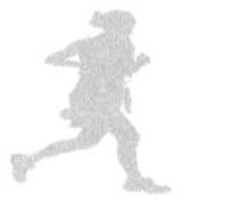 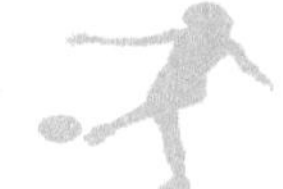 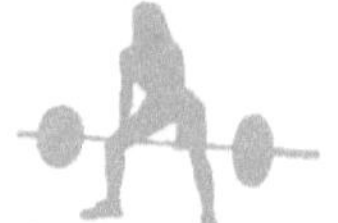 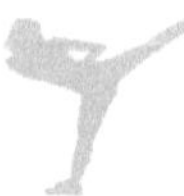 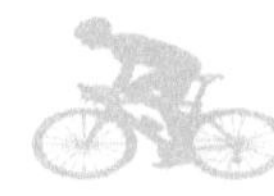

Cardio

ACTIVITY	DISTANCE	TIME	DONE

Weight Training

EXERCISE	SET ONE WEIGHT/REPS	SET TWO WEIGHT/REPS	SET THREE WEIGHT/REPS

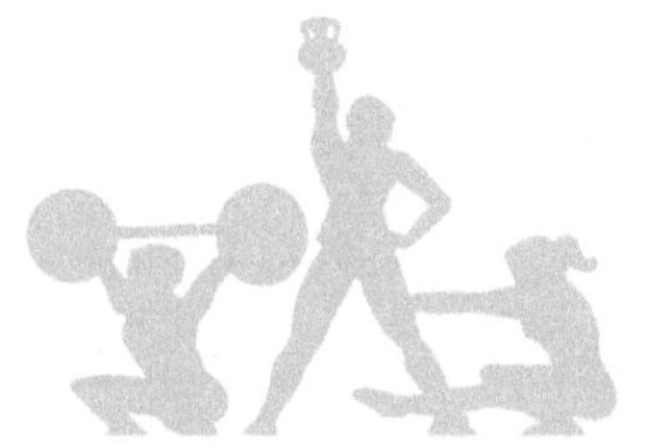

Name: ....

Date: ....

Time: ....

Warm-Up

ACTIVITY	TIME/REPS	DONE

 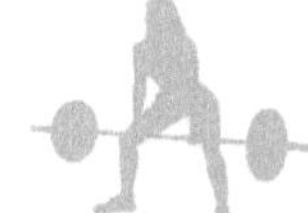 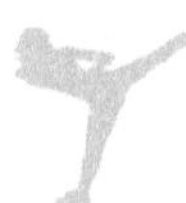 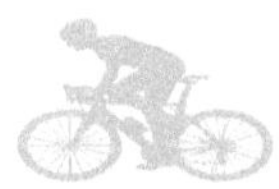

Cardio

ACTIVITY	DISTANCE	TIME	DONE

Weight Training

EXERCISE	SET ONE WEIGHT/REPS	SET TWO WEIGHT/REPS	SET THREE WEIGHT/REPS

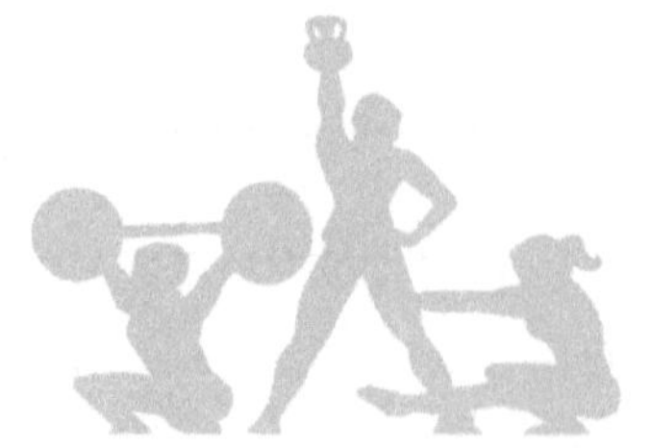

Name: ....

Date: ....

Time: ....

Warm-Up

ACTIVITY	TIME/REPS	DONE

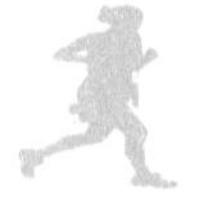  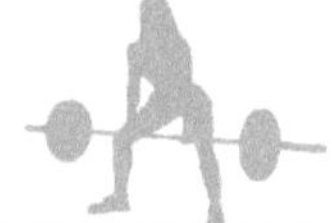 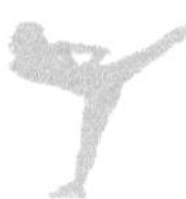 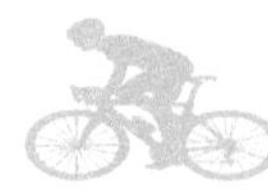

Cardio

ACTIVITY	DISTANCE	TIME	DONE

Weight Training

EXERCISE	SET ONE WEIGHT/REPS	SET TWO WEIGHT/REPS	SET THREE WEIGHT/REPS

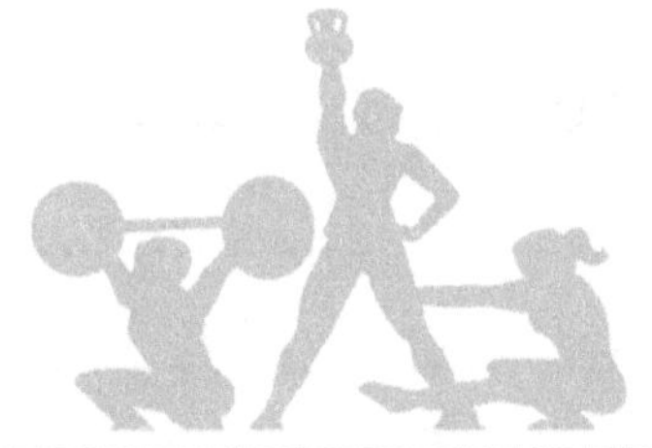

Name: ....

Date: ....

Time: ....

Warm-Up

ACTIVITY	TIME/REPS	DONE

 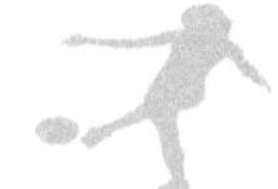 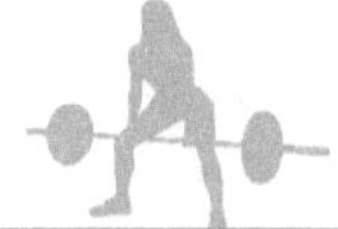 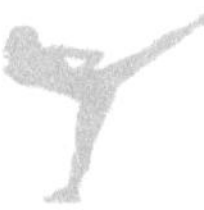 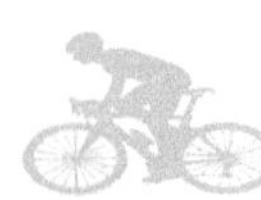

Cardio

ACTIVITY	DISTANCE	TIME	DONE

Weight Training

EXERCISE	SET ONE WEIGHT/REPS	SET TWO WEIGHT/REPS	SET THREE WEIGHT/REPS

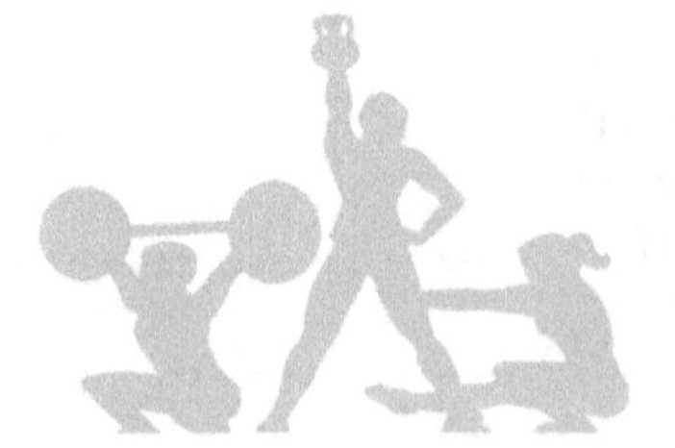

Warm-Up

ACTIVITY	TIME/REPS	DONE

 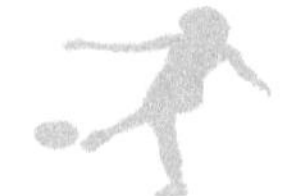 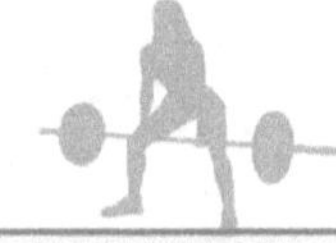 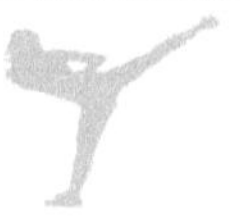 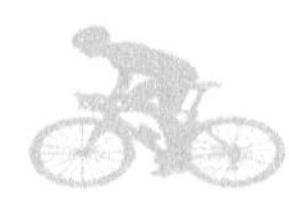

Cardio

ACTIVITY	DISTANCE	TIME	DONE

Weight Training

EXERCISE	SET ONE WEIGHT/REPS	SET TWO WEIGHT/REPS	SET THREE WEIGHT/REPS

Name: ....

Date: ....

Time: ....

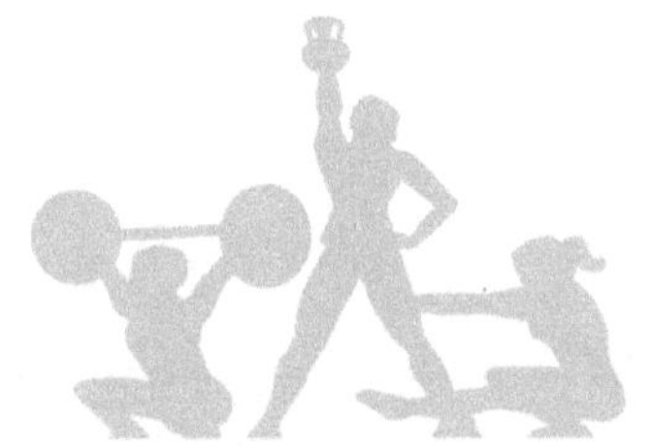

Name: ....

Date: ....

Time: ....

Warm-Up

ACTIVITY	TIME/REPS	DONE

 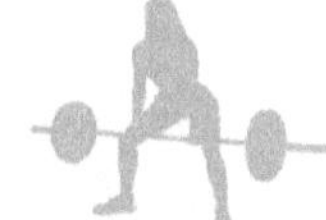 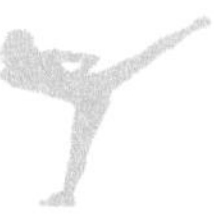 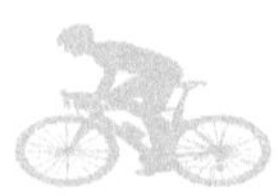

Cardio

ACTIVITY	DISTANCE	TIME	DONE

Weight Training

EXERCISE	SET ONE WEIGHT/REPS	SET TWO WEIGHT/REPS	SET THREE WEIGHT/REPS

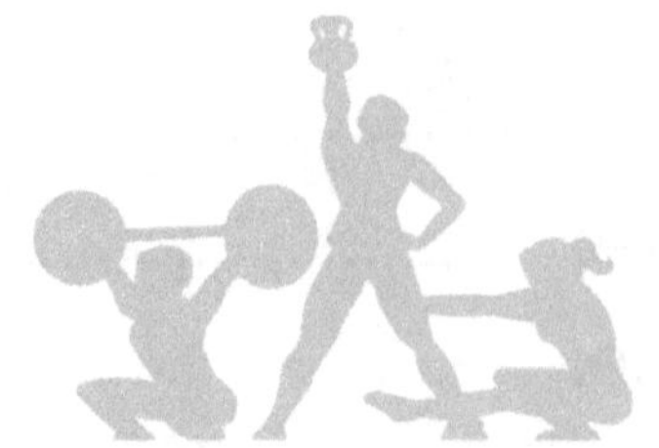

Name: ....

Date: ....

Time: ....

Warm-Up

ACTIVITY	TIME/REPS	DONE

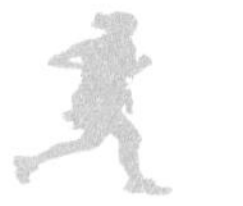 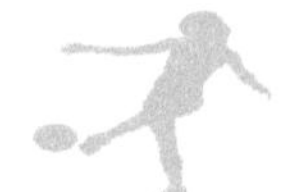 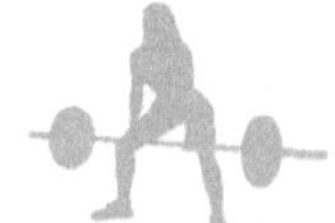 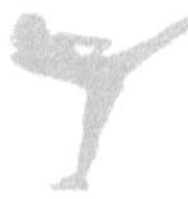 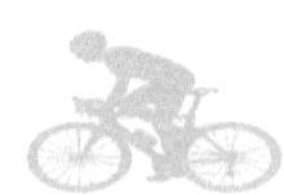

Cardio

ACTIVITY	DISTANCE	TIME	DONE

Weight Training

EXERCISE	SET ONE WEIGHT/REPS	SET TWO WEIGHT/REPS	SET THREE WEIGHT/REPS

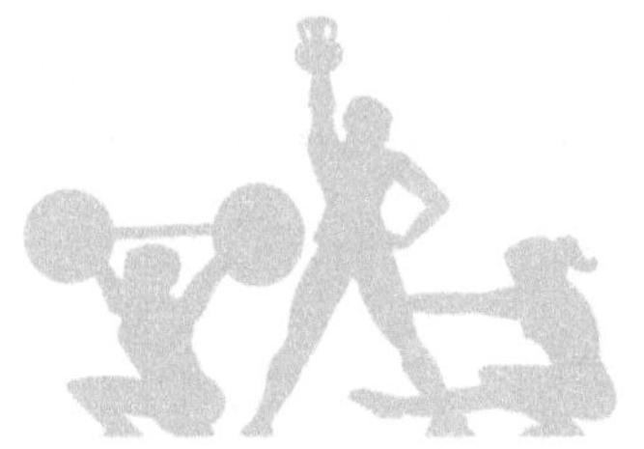

Name: ....

Date: ....

Time: ....

Warm-Up

ACTIVITY	TIME/REPS	DONE

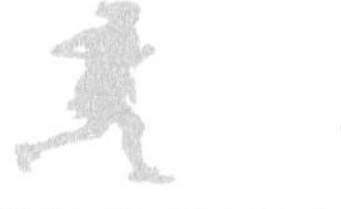 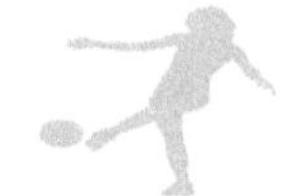 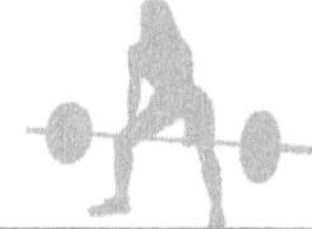 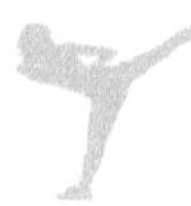 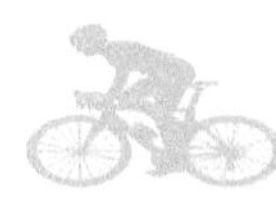

Cardio

ACTIVITY	DISTANCE	TIME	DONE

Weight Training

EXERCISE	SET ONE WEIGHT/REPS	SET TWO WEIGHT/REPS	SET THREE WEIGHT/REPS

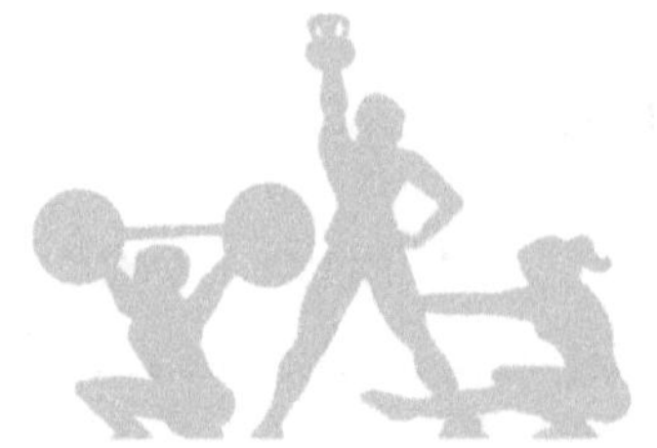

Name: ....

Date: ....

Time: ....

Warm-Up

ACTIVITY	TIME/REPS	DONE

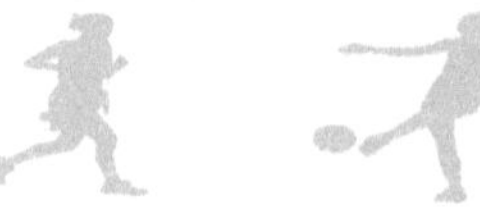 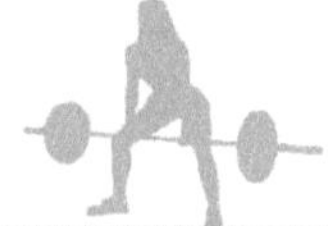 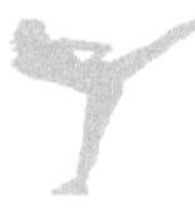 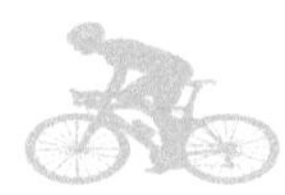

Cardio

ACTIVITY	DISTANCE	TIME	DONE

Weight Training

EXERCISE	SET ONE WEIGHT/REPS	SET TWO WEIGHT/REPS	SET THREE WEIGHT/REPS

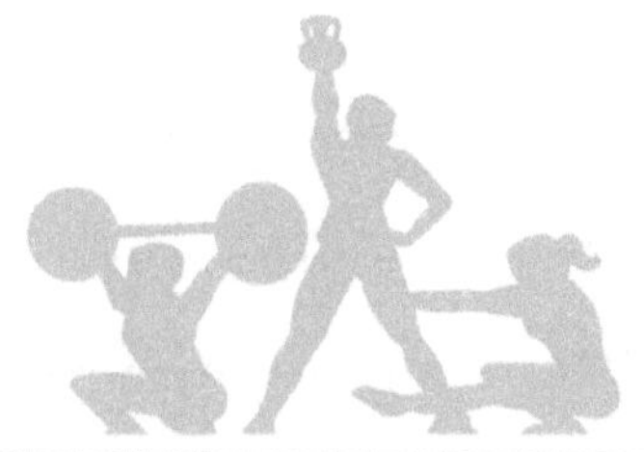

Name: ....

Date: ....

Time: ....

Warm-Up

ACTIVITY	TIME/REPS	DONE

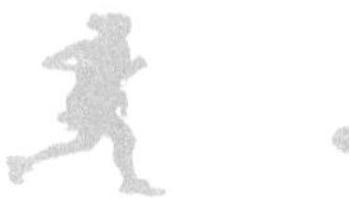 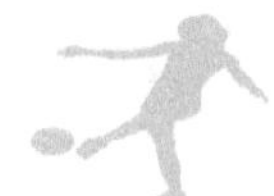 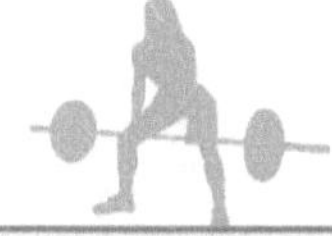 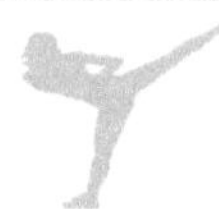 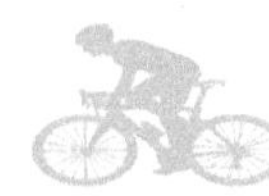

Cardio

ACTIVITY	DISTANCE	TIME	DONE

Weight Training

EXERCISE	SET ONE WEIGHT/REPS	SET TWO WEIGHT/REPS	SET THREE WEIGHT/REPS

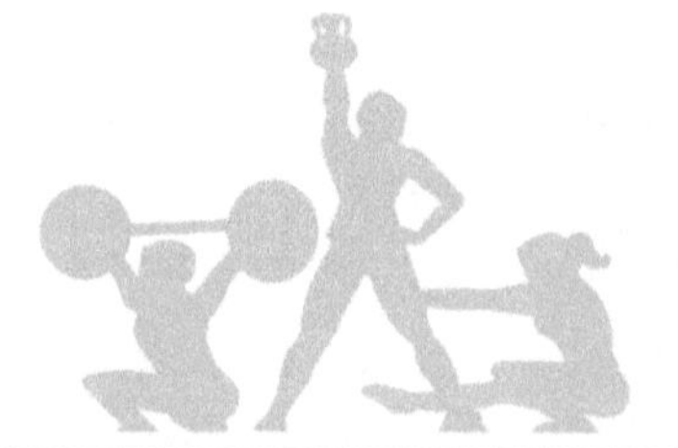

Name: ....

Date: ....

Time: ....

Warm-Up

ACTIVITY	TIME/REPS	DONE

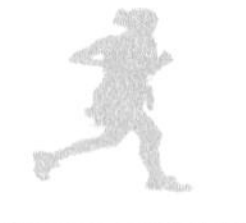 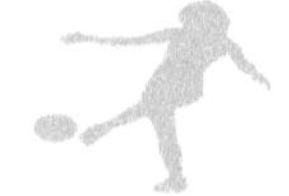 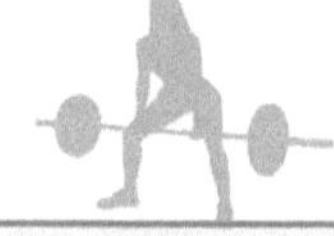 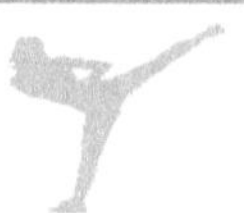 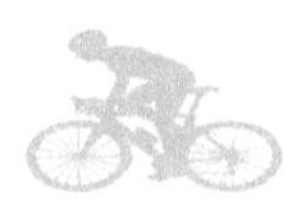

Cardio

ACTIVITY	DISTANCE	TIME	DONE

Weight Training

EXERCISE	SET ONE WEIGHT/REPS	SET TWO WEIGHT/REPS	SET THREE WEIGHT/REPS

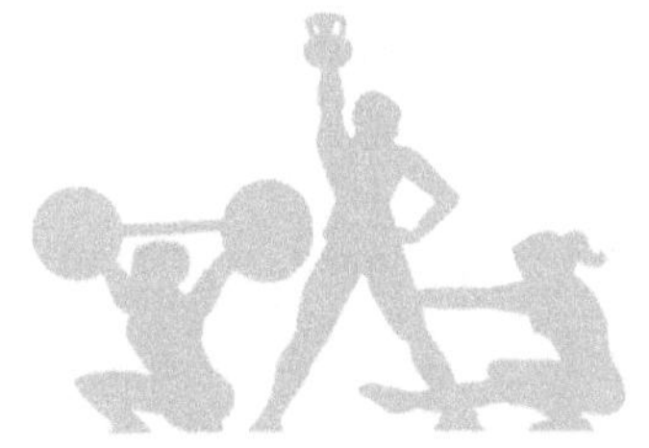

Name: ....

Date: ....

Time: ....

Warm-Up

ACTIVITY	TIME/REPS	DONE

 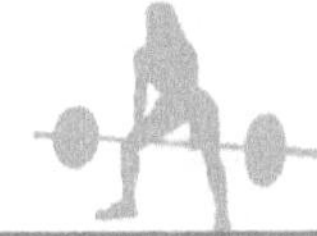 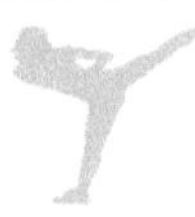 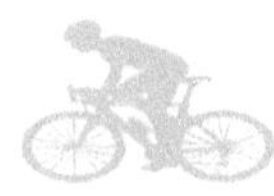

Cardio

ACTIVITY	DISTANCE	TIME	DONE

Weight Training

EXERCISE	SET ONE WEIGHT/REPS	SET TWO WEIGHT/REPS	SET THREE WEIGHT/REPS

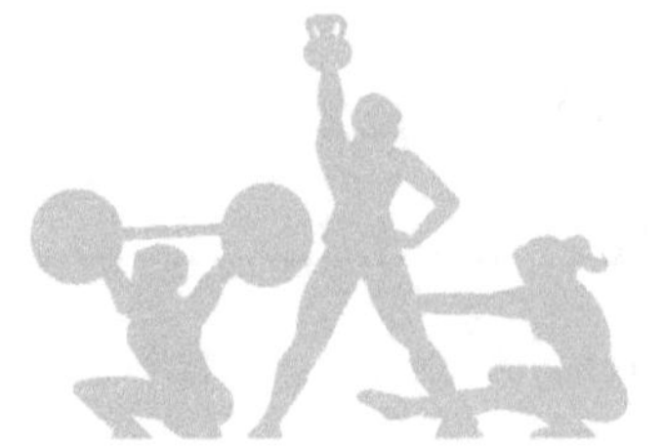

Name: ....

Date: ....

Time: ....

Warm-Up

ACTIVITY	TIME/REPS	DONE

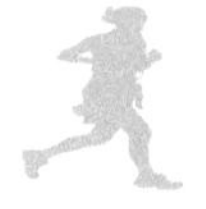 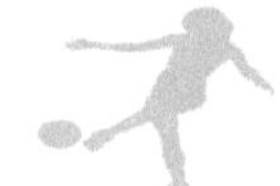 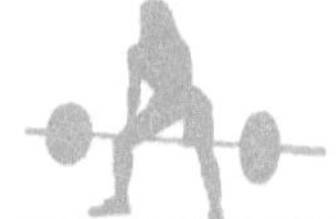 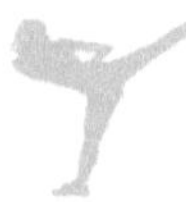 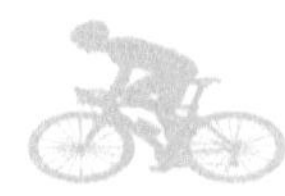

Cardio

ACTIVITY	DISTANCE	TIME	DONE

Weight Training

EXERCISE	SET ONE WEIGHT/REPS	SET TWO WEIGHT/REPS	SET THREE WEIGHT/REPS

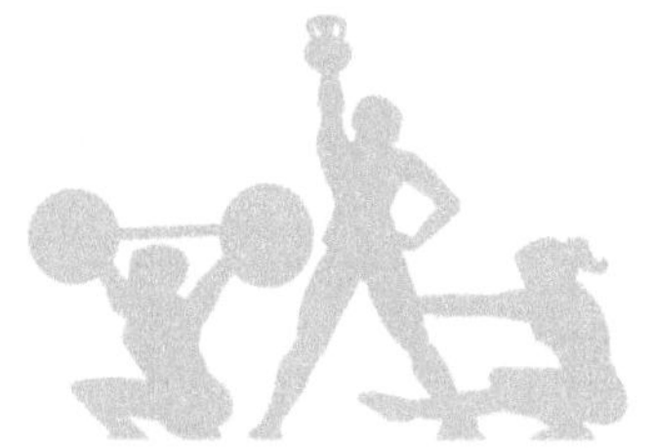

Name: ....

Date: ....

Time: ....

Warm-Up

ACTIVITY	TIME/REPS	DONE

 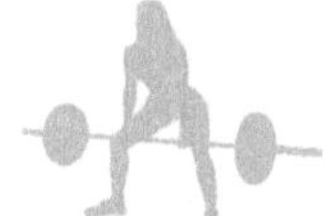 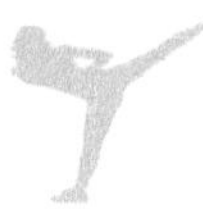 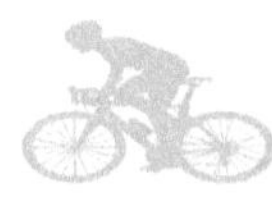

Cardio

ACTIVITY	DISTANCE	TIME	DONE

Weight Training

EXERCISE	SET ONE WEIGHT/REPS	SET TWO WEIGHT/REPS	SET THREE WEIGHT/REPS

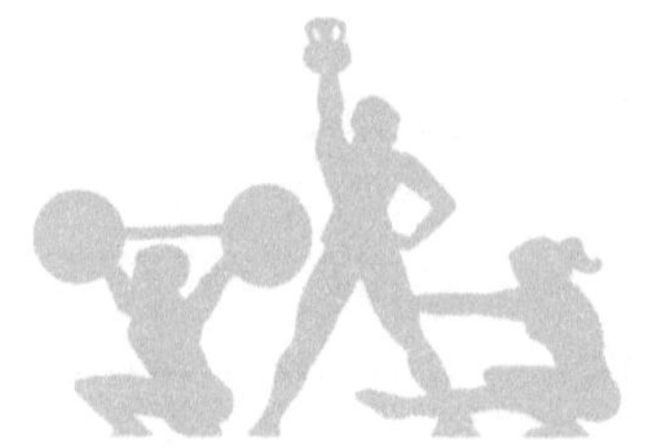

Name: ....

Date: ....

Time: ....

Warm-Up

ACTIVITY	TIME/REPS	DONE

 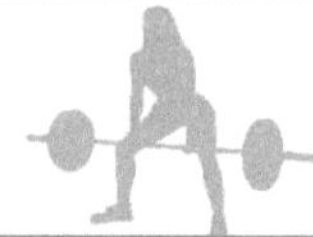 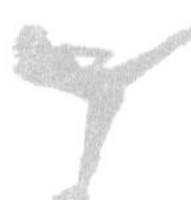 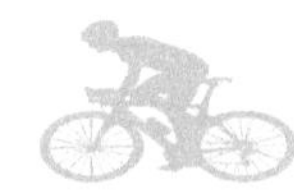

Cardio

ACTIVITY	DISTANCE	TIME	DONE

Weight Training

EXERCISE	SET ONE WEIGHT/REPS	SET TWO WEIGHT/REPS	SET THREE WEIGHT/REPS

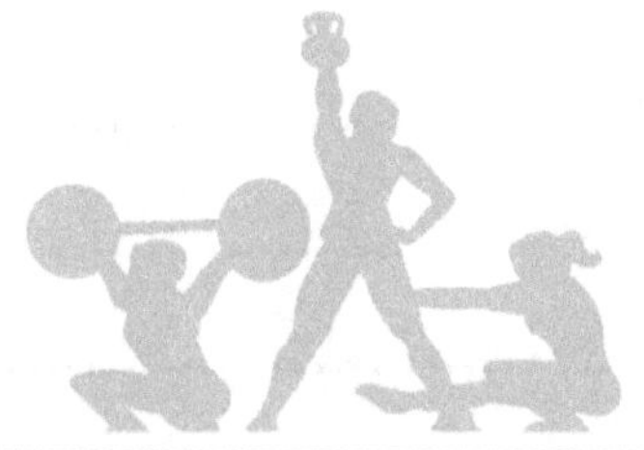

Name: ....

Date: ....

Time: ....

Warm-Up

ACTIVITY	TIME/REPS	DONE

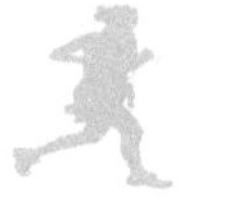 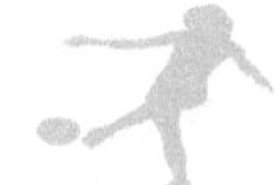 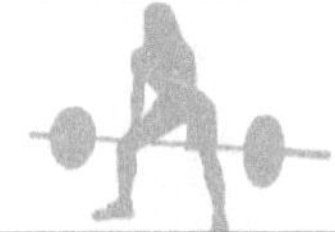 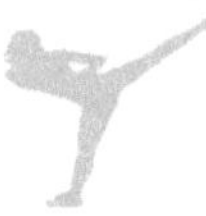 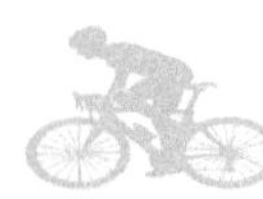

Cardio

ACTIVITY	DISTANCE	TIME	DONE

Weight Training

EXERCISE	SET ONE WEIGHT/REPS	SET TWO WEIGHT/REPS	SET THREE WEIGHT/REPS

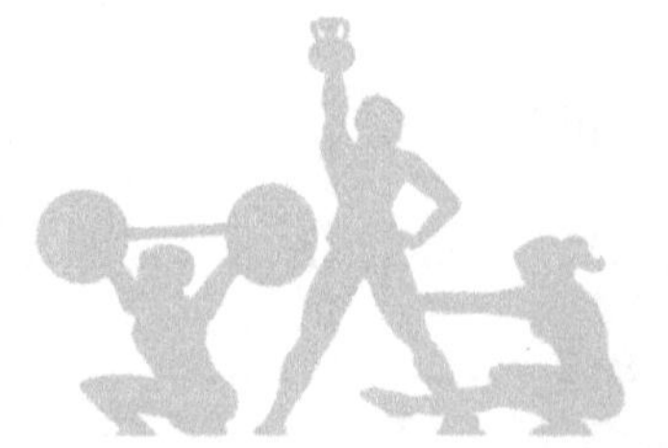

Name: ....

Date: ....

Time: ....

Warm-Up

ACTIVITY	TIME/REPS	DONE

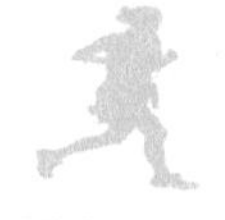 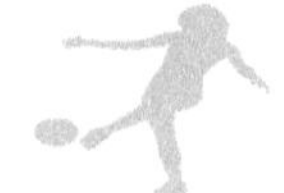 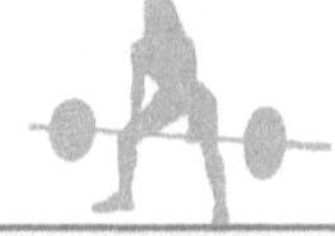 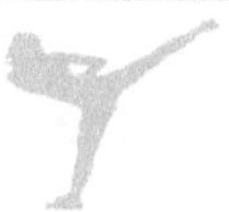 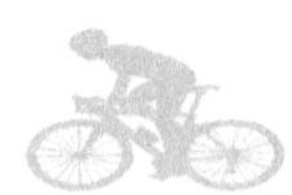

Cardio

ACTIVITY	DISTANCE	TIME	DONE

Weight Training

EXERCISE	SET ONE WEIGHT/REPS	SET TWO WEIGHT/REPS	SET THREE WEIGHT/REPS

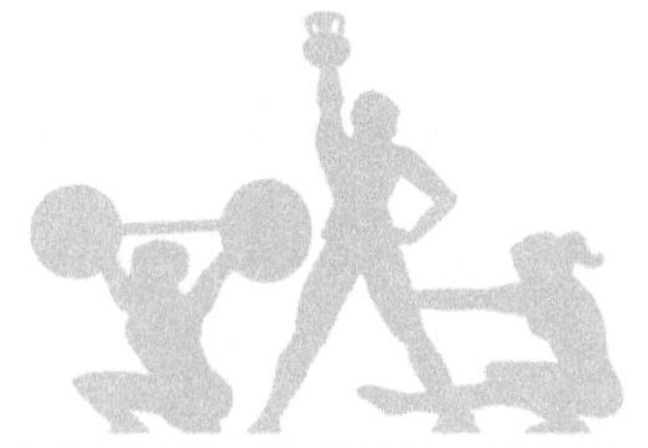

Name: ....

Date: ....

Time: ....

Warm-Up

ACTIVITY	TIME/REPS	DONE

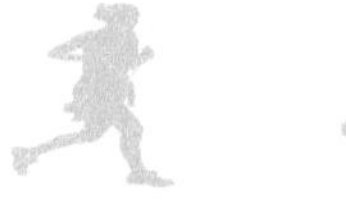 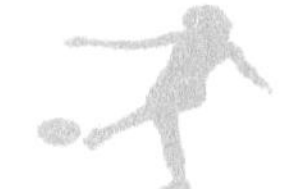 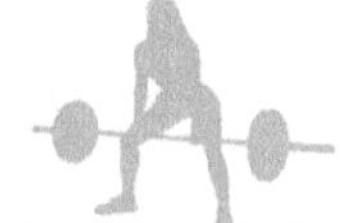 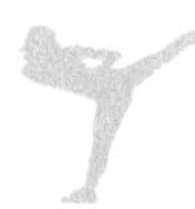 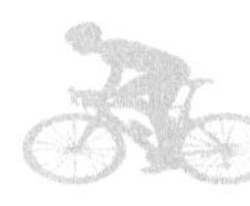

Cardio

ACTIVITY	DISTANCE	TIME	DONE

Weight Training

EXERCISE	SET ONE WEIGHT/REPS	SET TWO WEIGHT/REPS	SET THREE WEIGHT/REPS

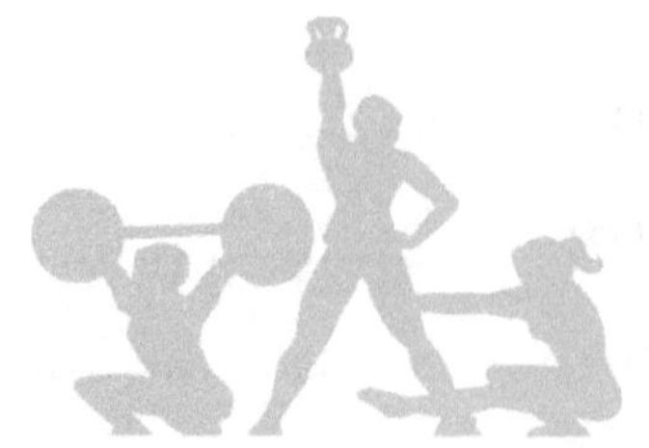

Warm-Up

ACTIVITY	TIME/REPS	DONE

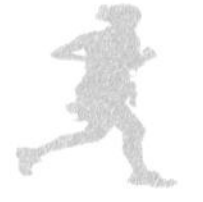 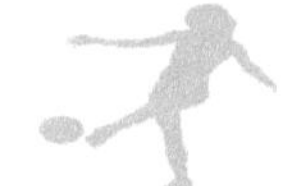 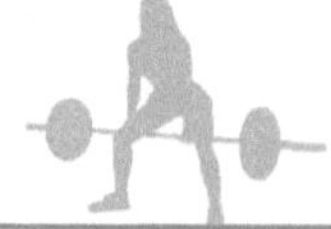 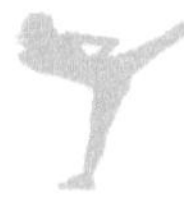 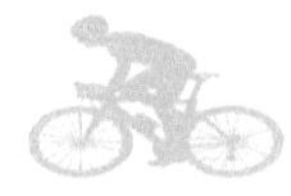

Cardio

ACTIVITY	DISTANCE	TIME	DONE

Weight Training

EXERCISE	SET ONE WEIGHT/REPS	SET TWO WEIGHT/REPS	SET THREE WEIGHT/REPS

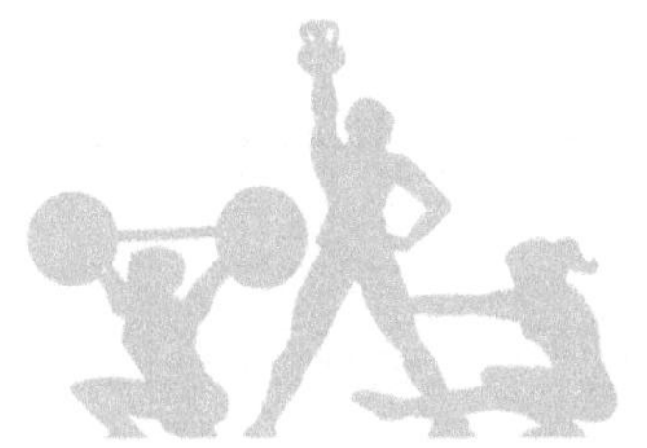

Name: ....

Date: ....

Time: ....

Warm-Up

ACTIVITY	TIME/REPS	DONE

 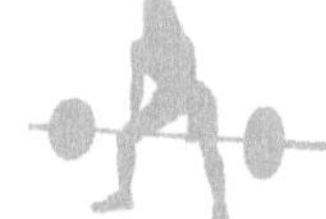 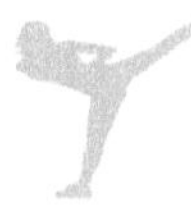 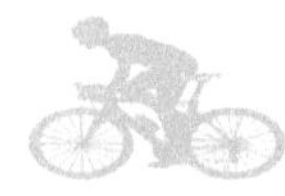

Cardio

ACTIVITY	DISTANCE	TIME	DONE

Weight Training

EXERCISE	SET ONE WEIGHT/REPS	SET TWO WEIGHT/REPS	SET THREE WEIGHT/REPS

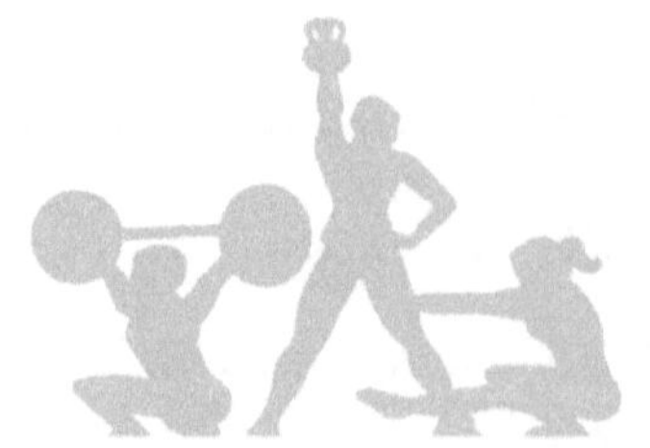

Name: ....

Date: ....

Time: ....

Warm-Up

ACTIVITY	TIME/REPS	DONE

 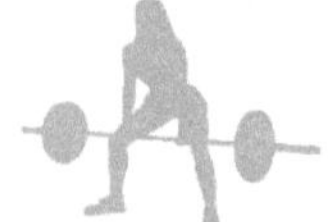 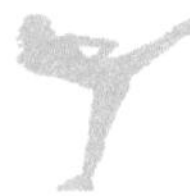 

Cardio

ACTIVITY	DISTANCE	TIME	DONE

Weight Training

EXERCISE	SET ONE WEIGHT/REPS	SET TWO WEIGHT/REPS	SET THREE WEIGHT/REPS

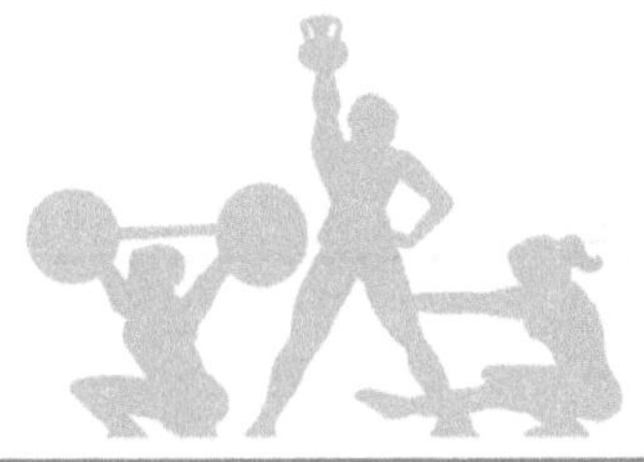

Name: ....

Date: ....

Time: ....

Warm-Up

ACTIVITY	TIME/REPS	DONE

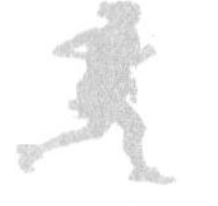 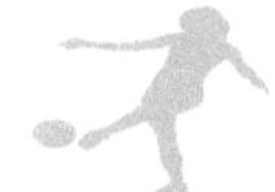 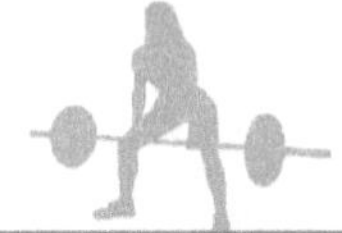 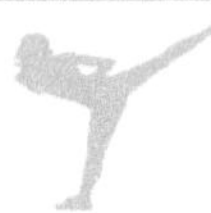 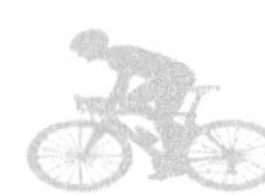

Cardio

ACTIVITY	DISTANCE	TIME	DONE

Weight Training

EXERCISE	SET ONE WEIGHT/REPS	SET TWO WEIGHT/REPS	SET THREE WEIGHT/REPS

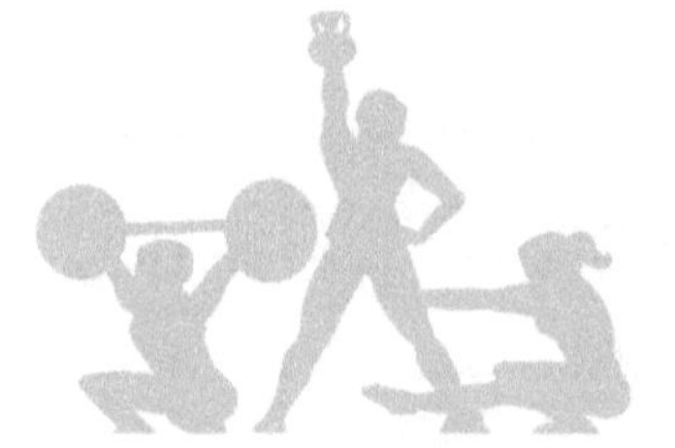

Name: ....

Date: ....

Time: ....

Warm-Up

ACTIVITY	TIME/REPS	DONE

 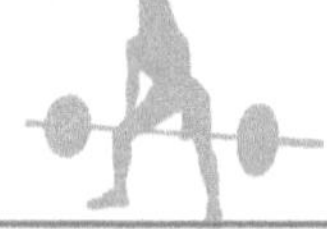 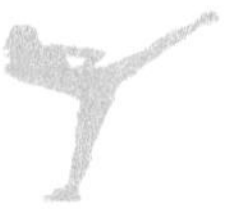 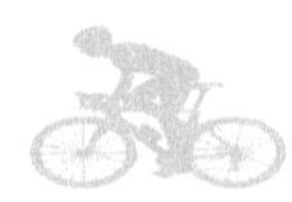

Cardio

ACTIVITY	DISTANCE	TIME	DONE

Weight Training

EXERCISE	SET ONE WEIGHT/REPS	SET TWO WEIGHT/REPS	SET THREE WEIGHT/REPS

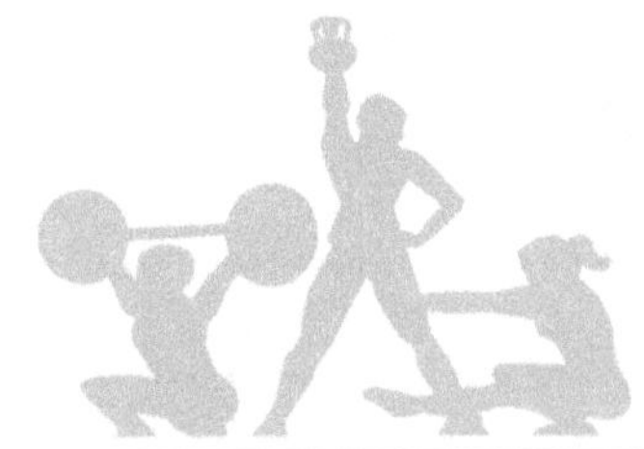

Name: ……………………………

Date: ……………………………

Time: ……………………………

Warm-Up

ACTIVITY	TIME/REPS	DONE

 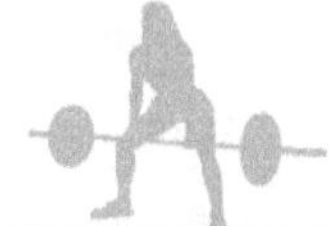 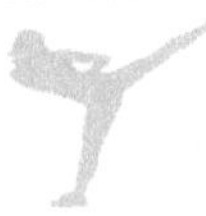 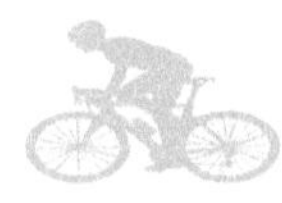

Cardio

ACTIVITY	DISTANCE	TIME	DONE

Weight Training

EXERCISE	SET ONE WEIGHT/REPS	SET TWO WEIGHT/REPS	SET THREE WEIGHT/REPS

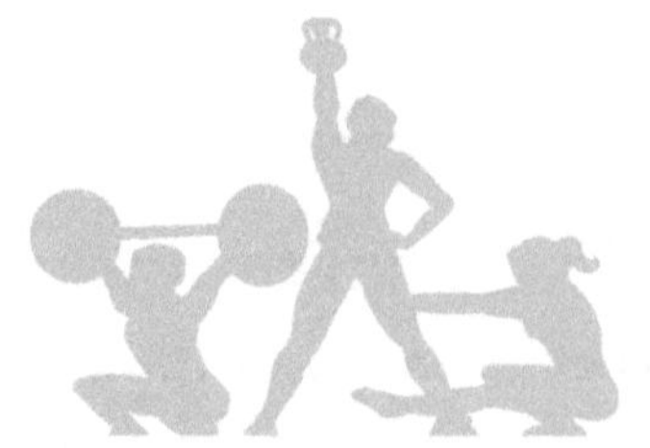

Name: ....

Date: ....

Time: ....

Warm-Up

ACTIVITY	TIME/REPS	DONE

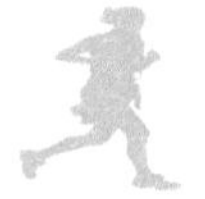 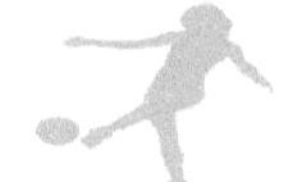 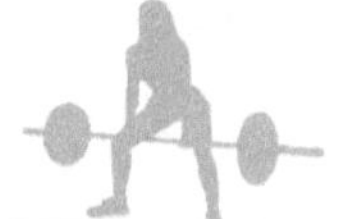 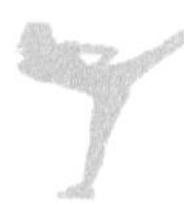 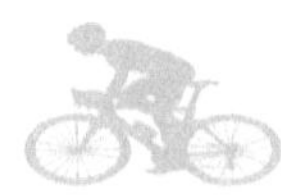

Cardio

ACTIVITY	DISTANCE	TIME	DONE

Weight Training

EXERCISE	SET ONE WEIGHT/REPS	SET TWO WEIGHT/REPS	SET THREE WEIGHT/REPS

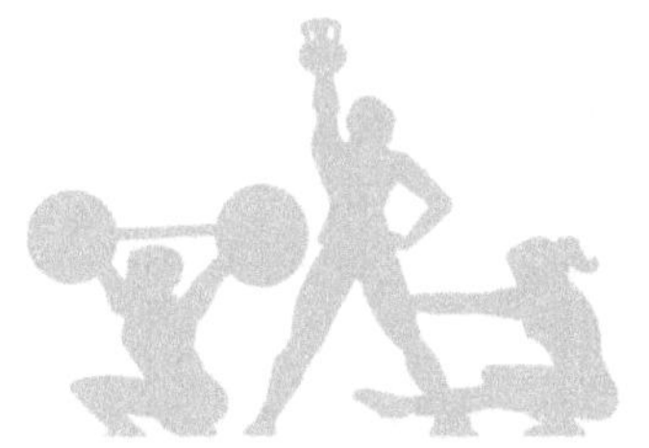

Name: ....

Date: ....

Time: ....

Warm-Up

ACTIVITY	TIME/REPS	DONE

  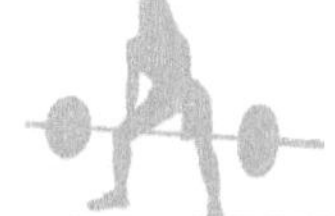 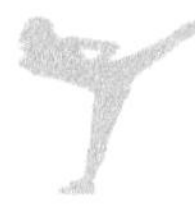 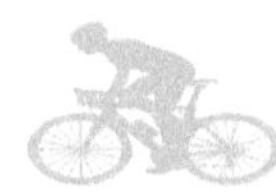

Cardio

ACTIVITY	DISTANCE	TIME	DONE

Weight Training

EXERCISE	SET ONE WEIGHT/REPS	SET TWO WEIGHT/REPS	SET THREE WEIGHT/REPS

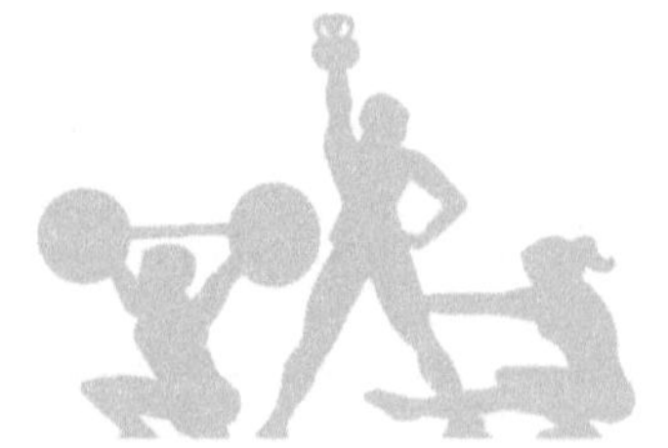

Name: ....

Date: ....

Time: ....

Warm-Up

ACTIVITY	TIME/REPS	DONE

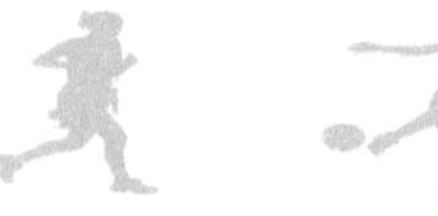 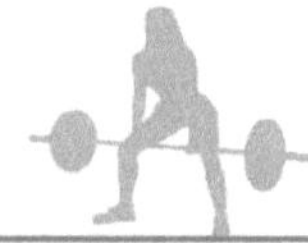 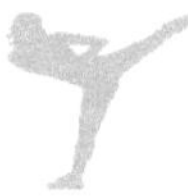 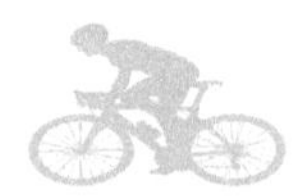

Cardio

ACTIVITY	DISTANCE	TIME	DONE

Weight Training

EXERCISE	SET ONE WEIGHT/REPS	SET TWO WEIGHT/REPS	SET THREE WEIGHT/REPS

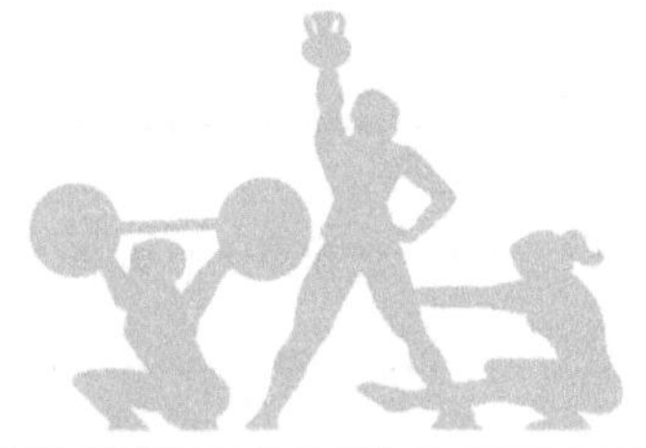

Name: ....

Date: ....

Time: ....

Warm-Up

ACTIVITY	TIME/REPS	DONE

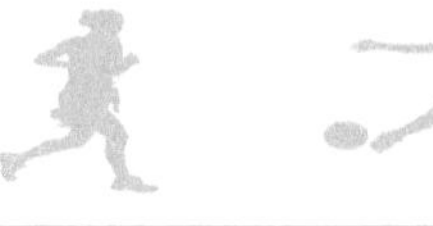 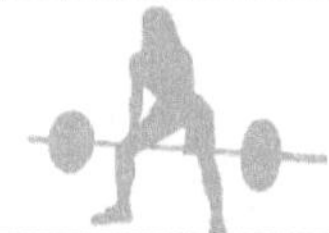 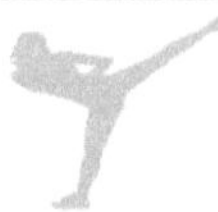 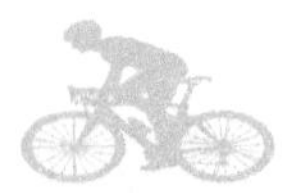

Cardio

ACTIVITY	DISTANCE	TIME	DONE

Weight Training

EXERCISE	SET ONE WEIGHT/REPS	SET TWO WEIGHT/REPS	SET THREE WEIGHT/REPS

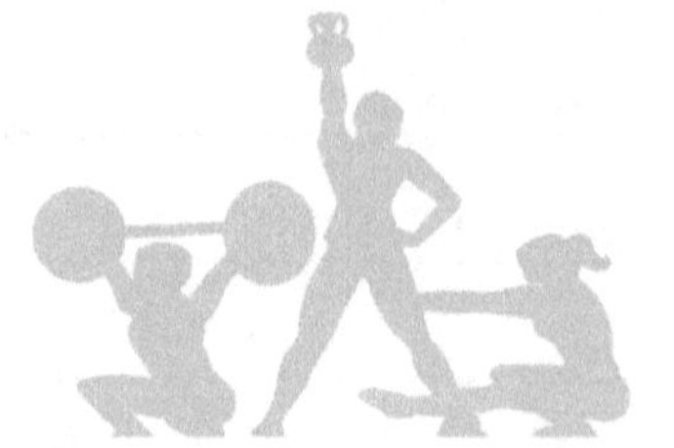

Warm-Up

ACTIVITY	TIME/REPS	DONE

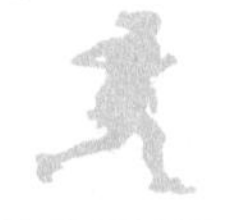 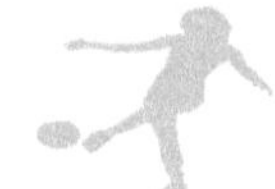 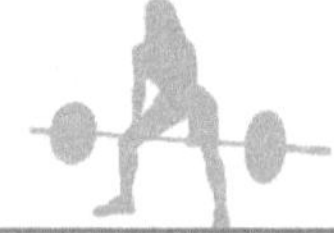 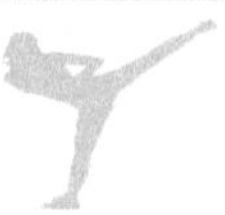 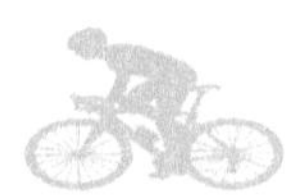

Cardio

ACTIVITY	DISTANCE	TIME	DONE

Weight Training

EXERCISE	SET ONE WEIGHT/REPS	SET TWO WEIGHT/REPS	SET THREE WEIGHT/REPS

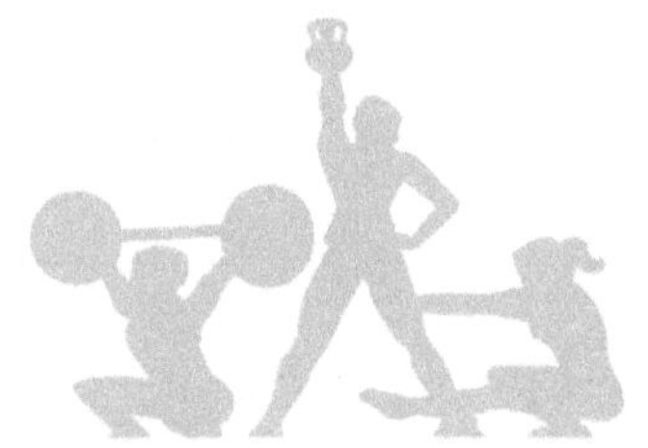

Name: ....

Date: ....

Time: ....

Warm-Up

ACTIVITY	TIME/REPS	DONE

 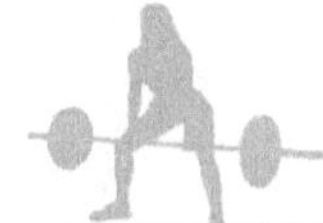 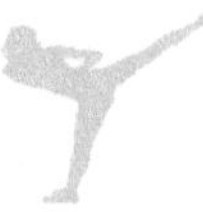 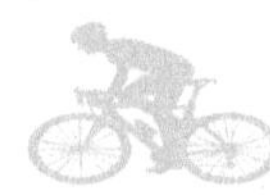

Cardio

ACTIVITY	DISTANCE	TIME	DONE

Weight Training

EXERCISE	SET ONE WEIGHT/REPS	SET TWO WEIGHT/REPS	SET THREE WEIGHT/REPS

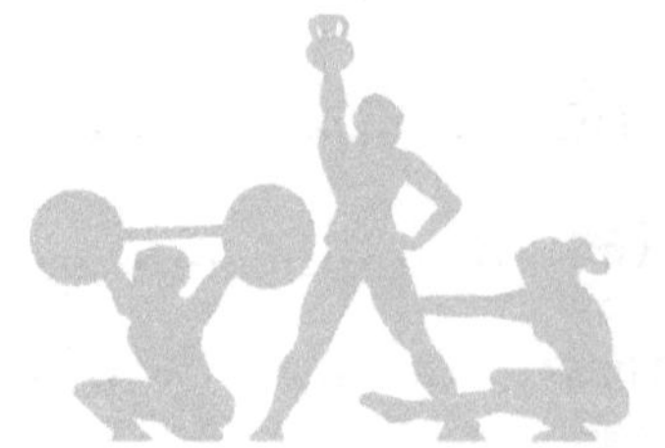

Name: ....

Date: ....

Time: ....

Warm-Up

ACTIVITY	TIME/REPS	DONE

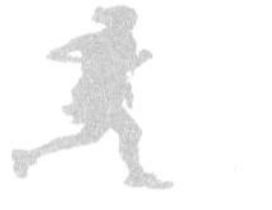 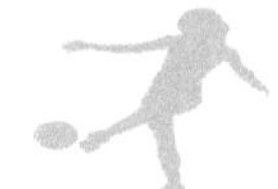 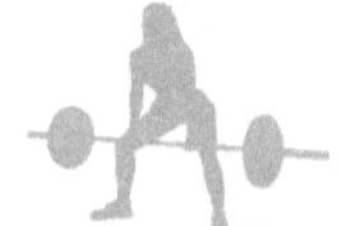 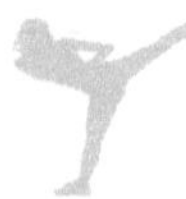 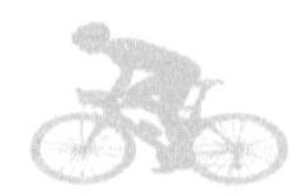

Cardio

ACTIVITY	DISTANCE	TIME	DONE

Weight Training

EXERCISE	SET ONE WEIGHT/REPS	SET TWO WEIGHT/REPS	SET THREE WEIGHT/REPS

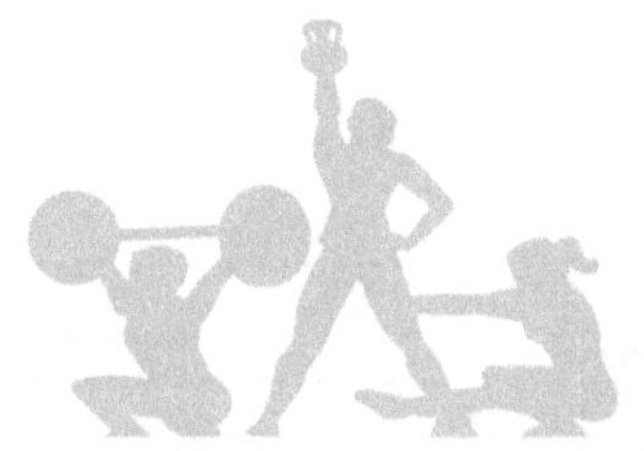

Name: ....

Date: ....

Time: ....

Warm-Up

ACTIVITY	TIME/REPS	DONE

 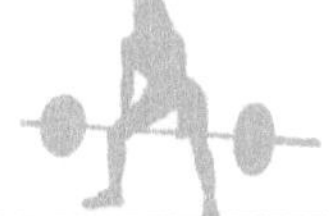 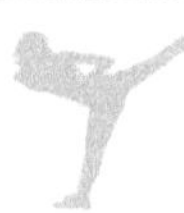 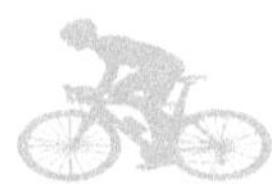

Cardio

ACTIVITY	DISTANCE	TIME	DONE

Weight Training

EXERCISE	SET ONE WEIGHT/REPS	SET TWO WEIGHT/REPS	SET THREE WEIGHT/REPS

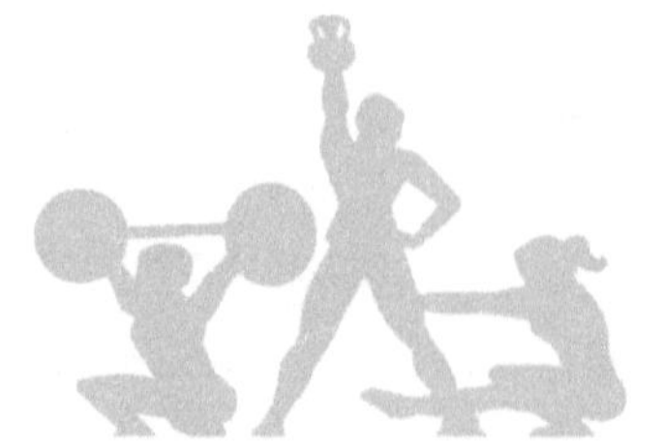

Name: ....

Date: ....

Time: ....

Warm-Up

ACTIVITY	TIME/REPS	DONE

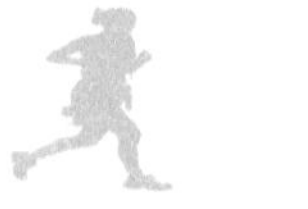 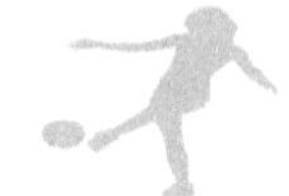 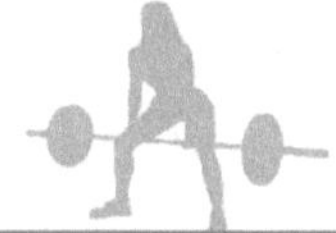 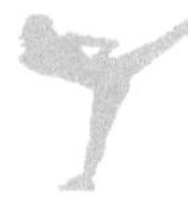 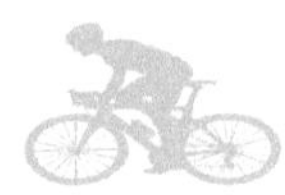

Cardio

ACTIVITY	DISTANCE	TIME	DONE

Weight Training

EXERCISE	SET ONE WEIGHT/REPS	SET TWO WEIGHT/REPS	SET THREE WEIGHT/REPS

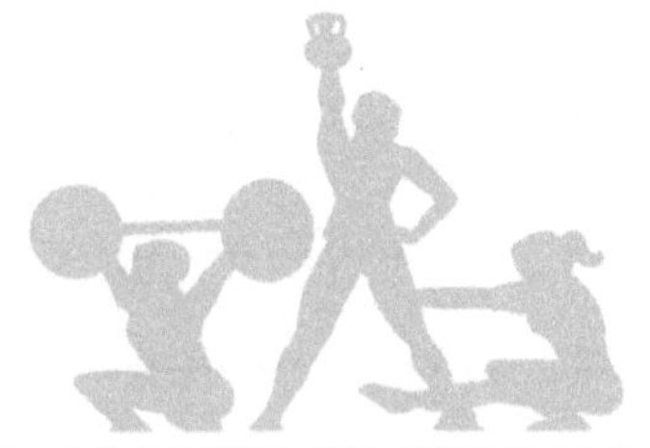

Warm-Up

ACTIVITY	TIME/REPS	DONE

  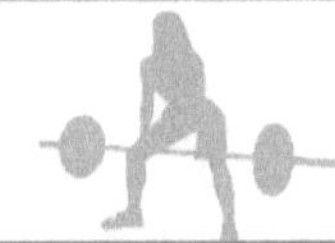 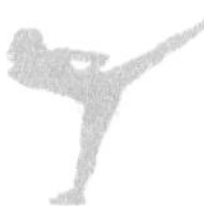 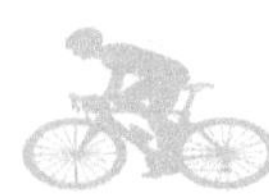

Cardio

ACTIVITY	DISTANCE	TIME	DONE

Weight Training

EXERCISE	SET ONE WEIGHT/REPS	SET TWO WEIGHT/REPS	SET THREE WEIGHT/REPS

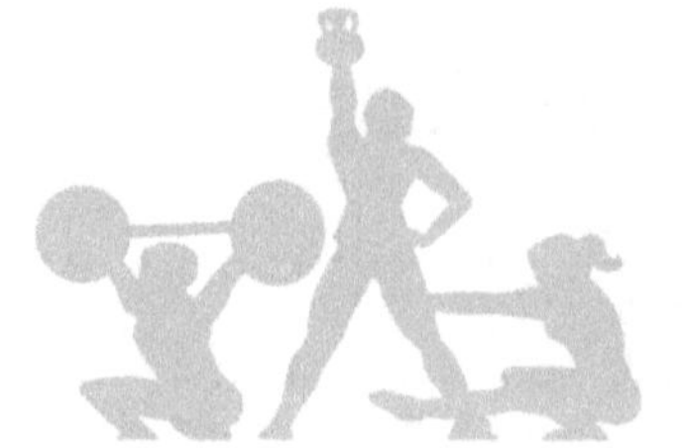

Name: ....

Date: ....

Time: ....

Warm-Up

ACTIVITY	TIME/REPS	DONE

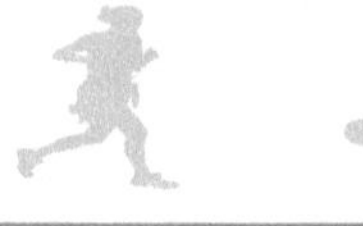 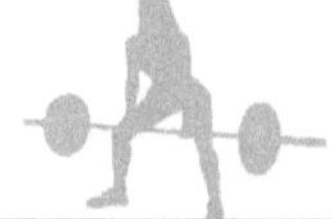 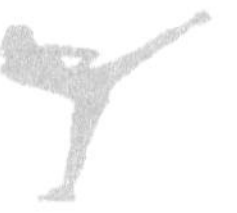 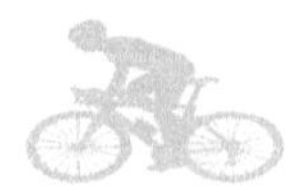

Cardio

ACTIVITY	DISTANCE	TIME	DONE

Weight Training

EXERCISE	SET ONE WEIGHT/REPS	SET TWO WEIGHT/REPS	SET THREE WEIGHT/REPS

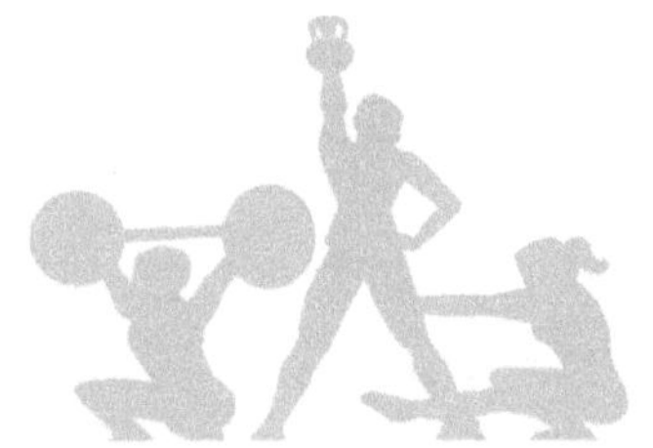

Warm-Up

ACTIVITY	TIME/REPS	DONE

 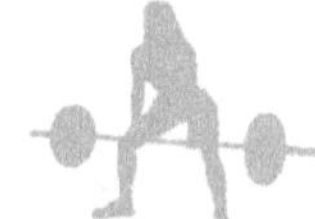 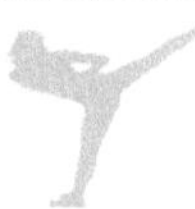 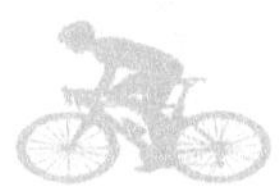

Cardio

ACTIVITY	DISTANCE	TIME	DONE

Weight Training

EXERCISE	SET ONE WEIGHT/REPS	SET TWO WEIGHT/REPS	SET THREE WEIGHT/REPS

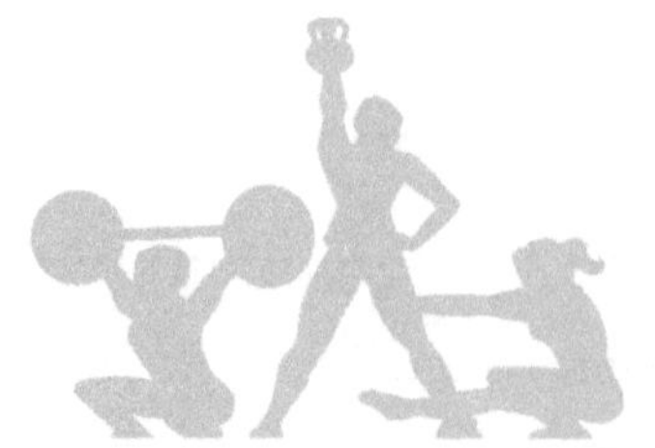

Name: ....

Date: ....

Time: ....

Warm-Up

ACTIVITY	TIME/REPS	DONE

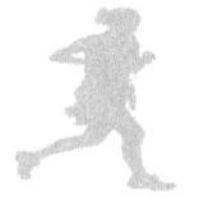 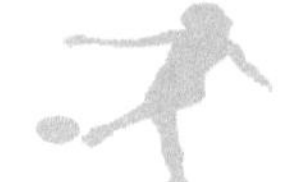 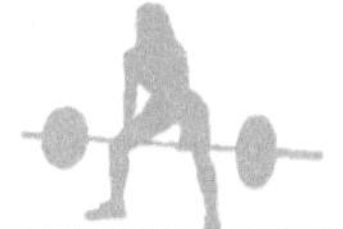 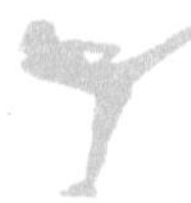 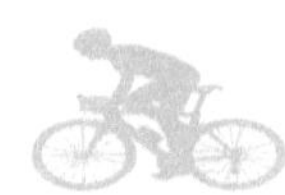

Cardio

ACTIVITY	DISTANCE	TIME	DONE

Weight Training

EXERCISE	SET ONE WEIGHT/REPS	SET TWO WEIGHT/REPS	SET THREE WEIGHT/REPS

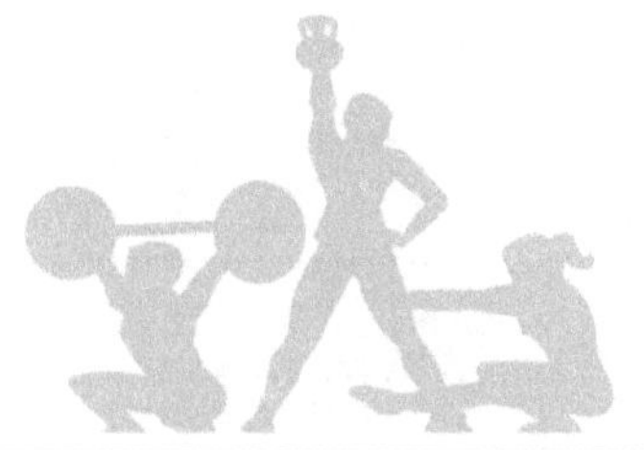

Name: ……………………………

Date: ……………………………

Time: ……………………………

Warm-Up

ACTIVITY	TIME/REPS	DONE

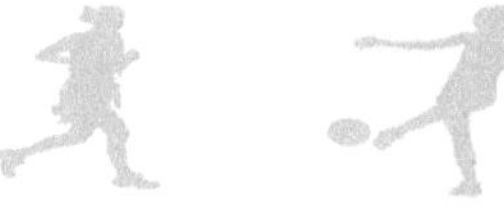 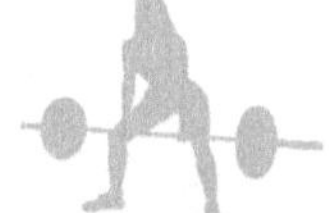 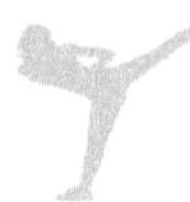 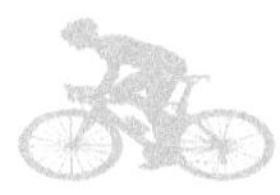

Cardio

ACTIVITY	DISTANCE	TIME	DONE

Weight Training

EXERCISE	SET ONE WEIGHT/REPS	SET TWO WEIGHT/REPS	SET THREE WEIGHT/REPS

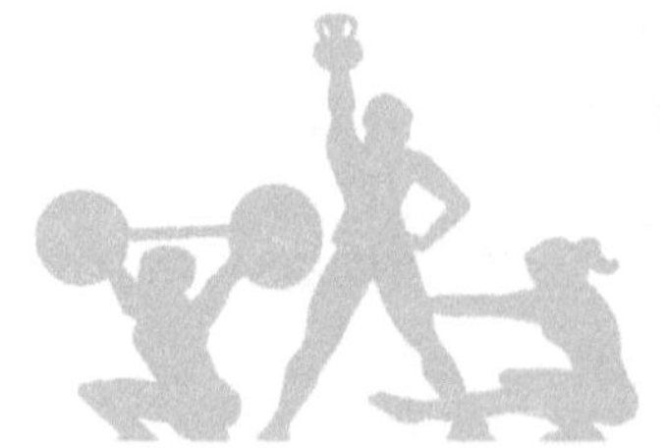

Name: ....

Date: ....

Time: ....

Warm-Up

ACTIVITY	TIME/REPS	DONE

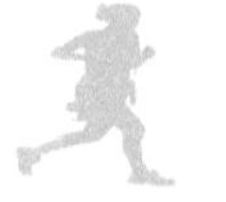 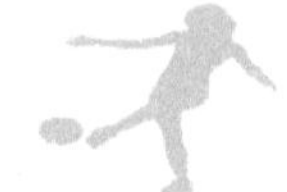 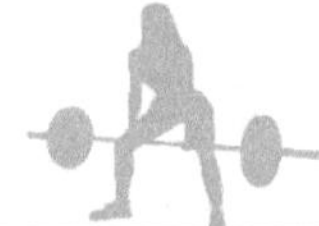 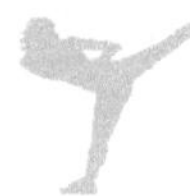 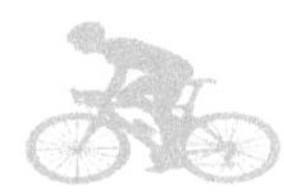

Cardio

ACTIVITY	DISTANCE	TIME	DONE

Weight Training

EXERCISE	SET ONE WEIGHT/REPS	SET TWO WEIGHT/REPS	SET THREE WEIGHT/REPS

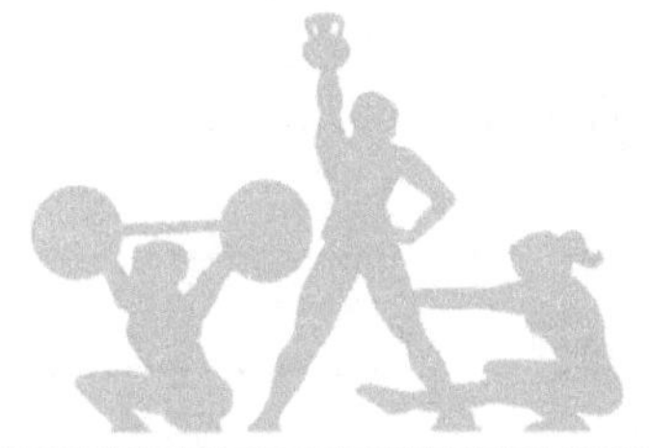

Name: ....

Date: ....

Time: ....

Warm-Up

ACTIVITY	TIME/REPS	DONE

 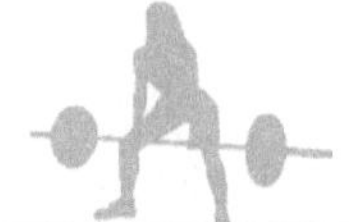 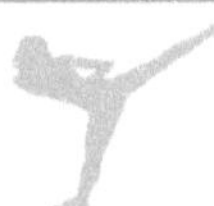 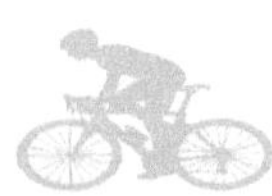

Cardio

ACTIVITY	DISTANCE	TIME	DONE

Weight Training

EXERCISE	SET ONE WEIGHT/REPS	SET TWO WEIGHT/REPS	SET THREE WEIGHT/REPS

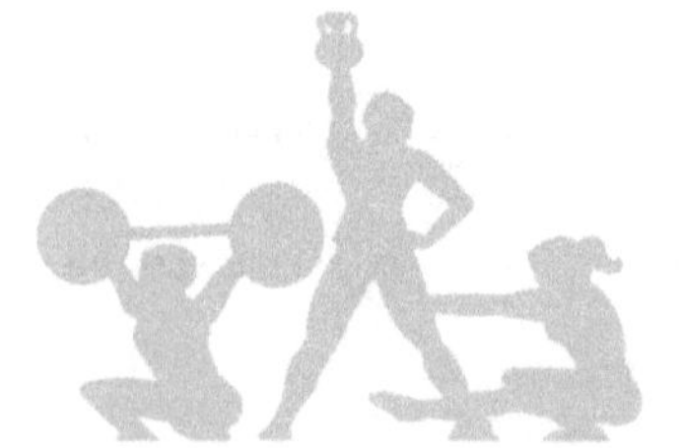

Name: ....

Date: ....

Time: ....

Warm-Up

ACTIVITY	TIME/REPS	DONE

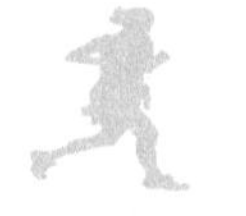 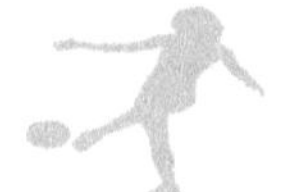 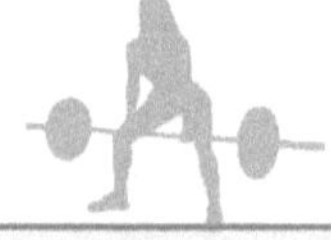 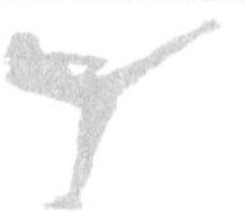 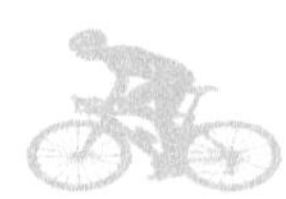

Cardio

ACTIVITY	DISTANCE	TIME	DONE

Weight Training

EXERCISE	SET ONE WEIGHT/REPS	SET TWO WEIGHT/REPS	SET THREE WEIGHT/REPS

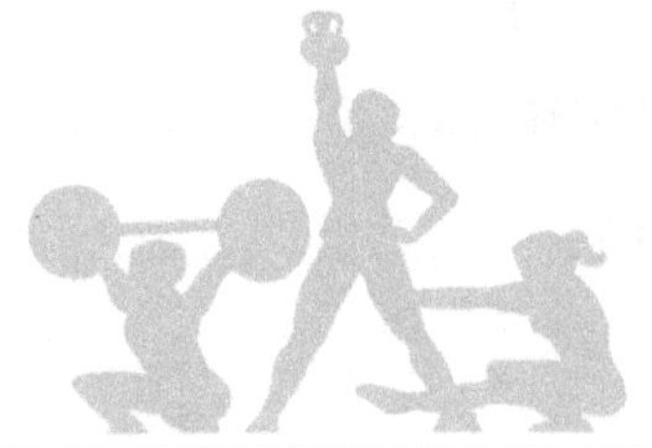

Name: ....

Date: ....

Time: ....

Warm-Up

ACTIVITY	TIME/REPS	DONE

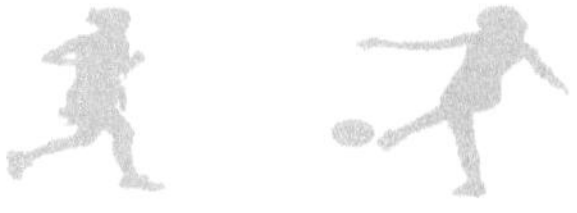 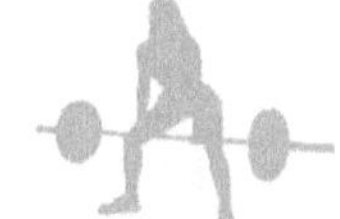 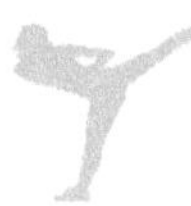 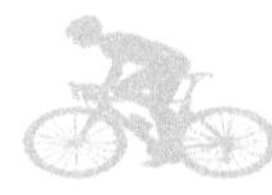

Cardio

ACTIVITY	DISTANCE	TIME	DONE

Weight Training

EXERCISE	SET ONE WEIGHT/REPS	SET TWO WEIGHT/REPS	SET THREE WEIGHT/REPS

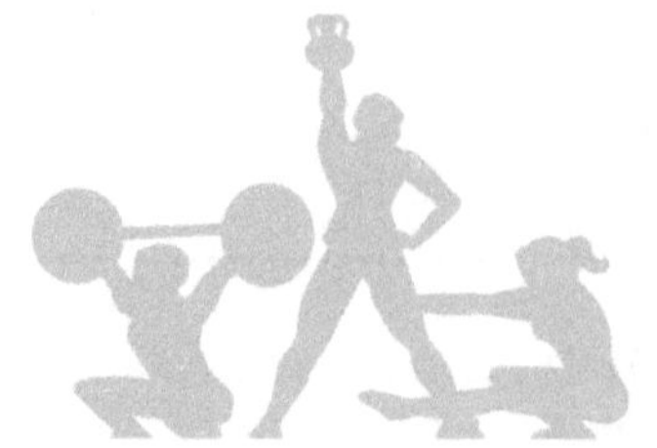

Name: ....

Date: ....

Time: ....

Warm-Up

ACTIVITY	TIME/REPS	DONE

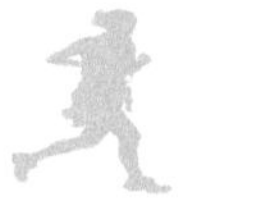 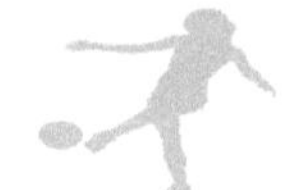 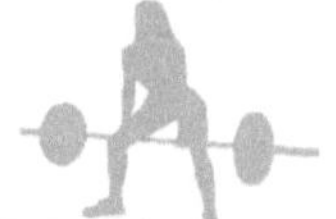 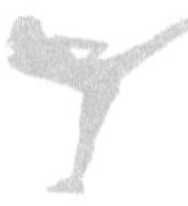 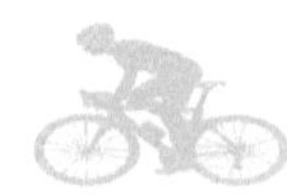

Cardio

ACTIVITY	DISTANCE	TIME	DONE

Weight Training

EXERCISE	SET ONE WEIGHT/REPS	SET TWO WEIGHT/REPS	SET THREE WEIGHT/REPS

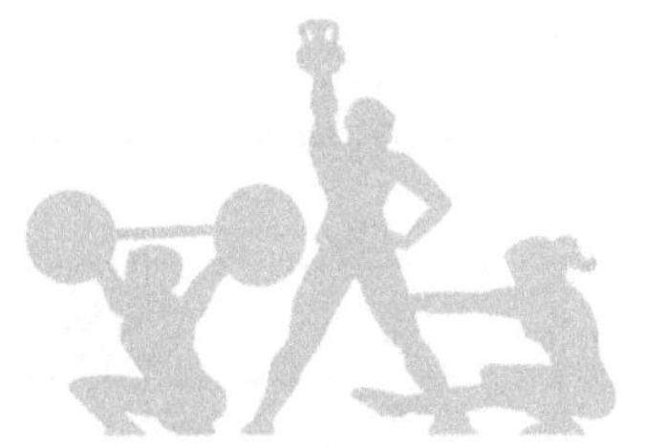

Warm-Up

ACTIVITY	TIME/REPS	DONE

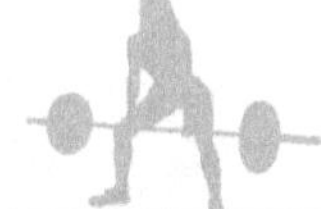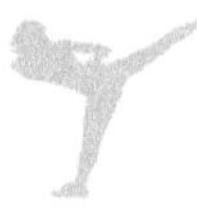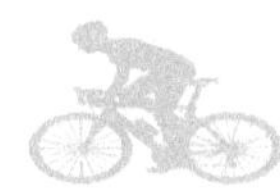

Cardio

ACTIVITY	DISTANCE	TIME	DONE

Weight Training

EXERCISE	SET ONE WEIGHT/REPS	SET TWO WEIGHT/REPS	SET THREE WEIGHT/REPS

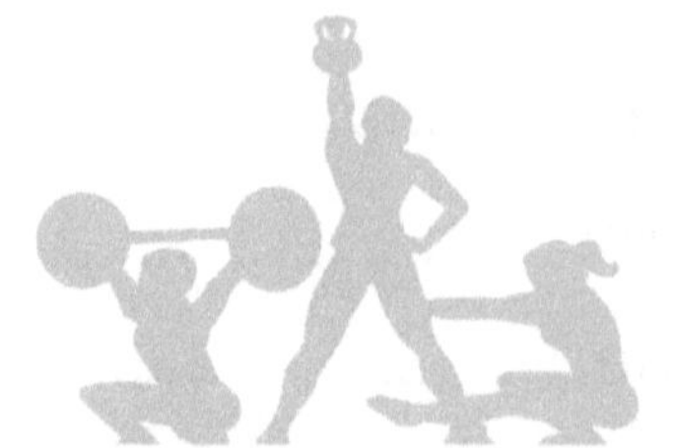

Warm-Up

ACTIVITY	TIME/REPS	DONE

 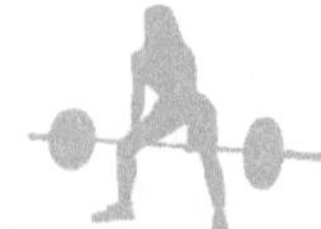 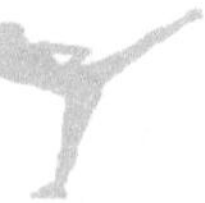 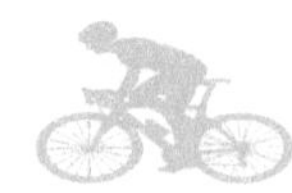

Cardio

ACTIVITY	DISTANCE	TIME	DONE

Weight Training

EXERCISE	SET ONE WEIGHT/REPS	SET TWO WEIGHT/REPS	SET THREE WEIGHT/REPS

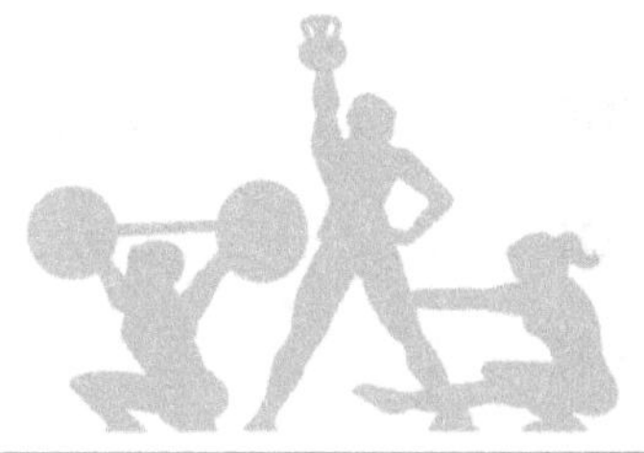

Name: ....

Date: ....

Time: ....

Warm-Up

ACTIVITY	TIME/REPS	DONE

 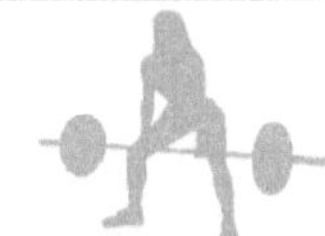 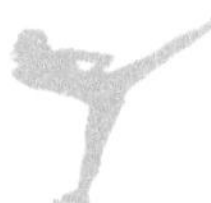 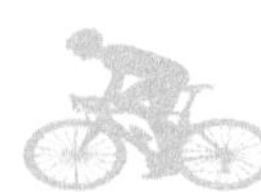

Cardio

ACTIVITY	DISTANCE	TIME	DONE

Weight Training

EXERCISE	SET ONE WEIGHT/REPS	SET TWO WEIGHT/REPS	SET THREE WEIGHT/REPS

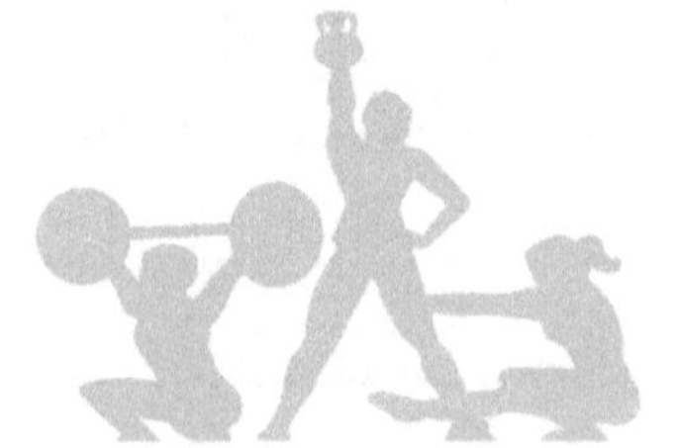

Name: ....

Date: ....

Time: ....

Warm-Up

ACTIVITY	TIME/REPS	DONE

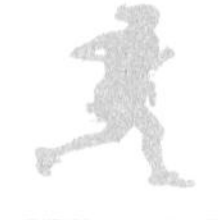 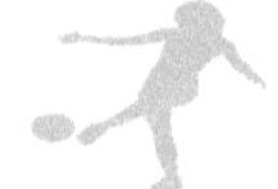 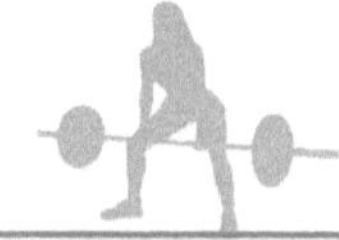 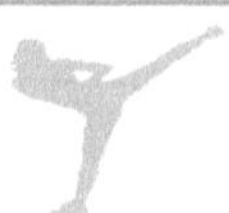 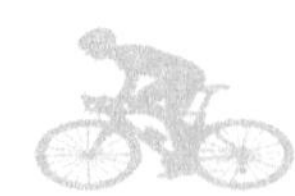

Cardio

ACTIVITY	DISTANCE	TIME	DONE

Weight Training

EXERCISE	SET ONE WEIGHT/REPS	SET TWO WEIGHT/REPS	SET THREE WEIGHT/REPS

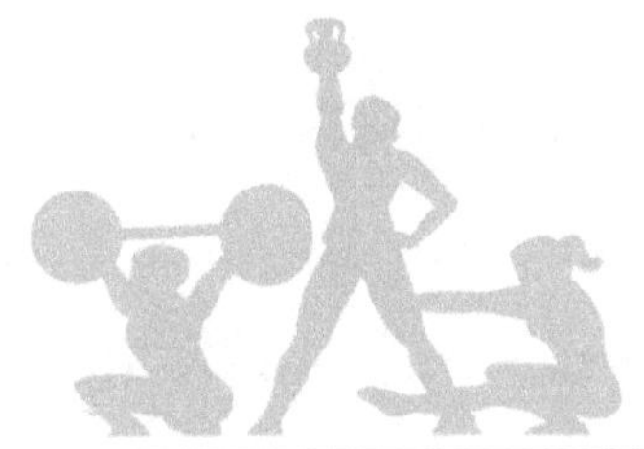

Name: ....

Date: ....

Time: ....

Warm-Up

ACTIVITY	TIME/REPS	DONE

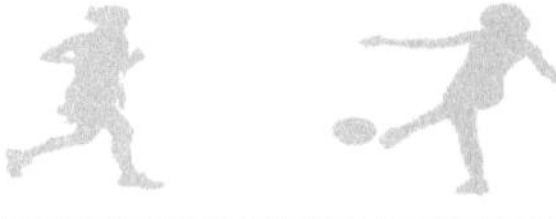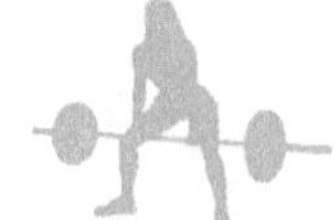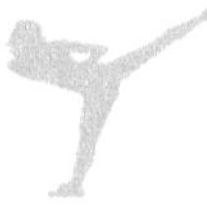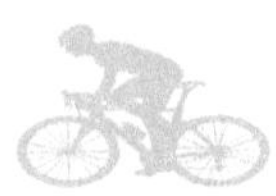

Cardio

ACTIVITY	DISTANCE	TIME	DONE

Weight Training

EXERCISE	SET ONE WEIGHT/REPS	SET TWO WEIGHT/REPS	SET THREE WEIGHT/REPS

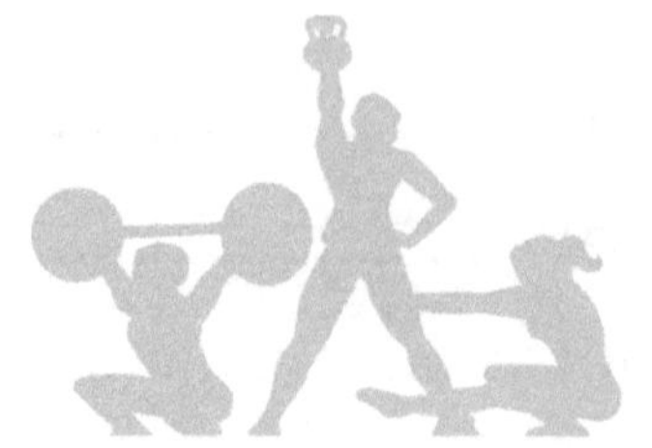

Name: ....

Date: ....

Time: ....

Warm-Up

ACTIVITY	TIME/REPS	DONE

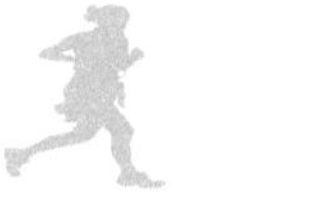 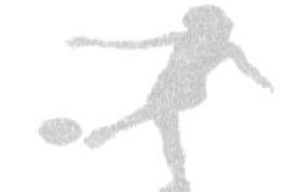 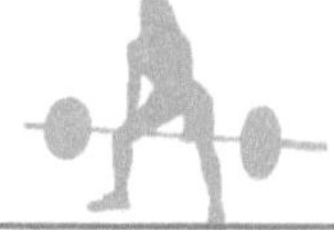 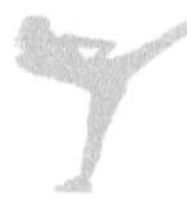 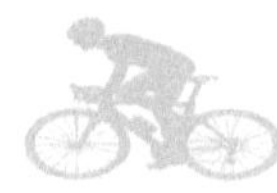

Cardio

ACTIVITY	DISTANCE	TIME	DONE

Weight Training

EXERCISE	SET ONE WEIGHT/REPS	SET TWO WEIGHT/REPS	SET THREE WEIGHT/REPS

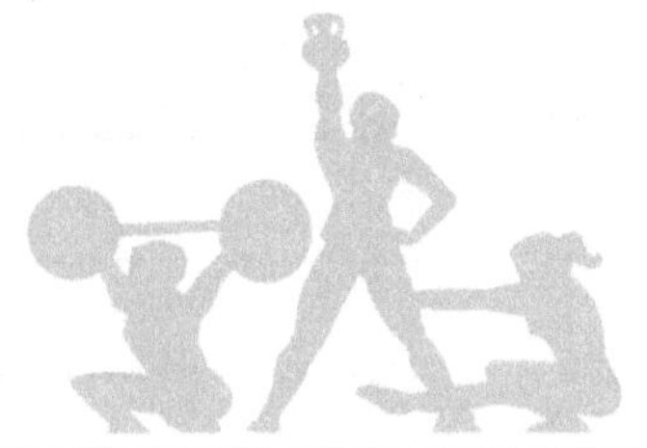

Name: ....

Date: ....

Time: ....

Warm-Up

ACTIVITY	TIME/REPS	DONE

 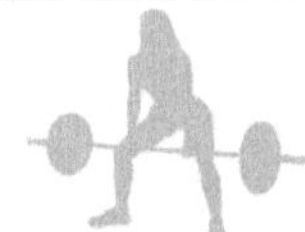 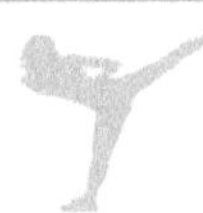 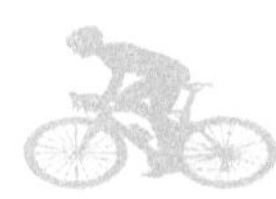

Cardio

ACTIVITY	DISTANCE	TIME	DONE

Weight Training

EXERCISE	SET ONE WEIGHT/REPS	SET TWO WEIGHT/REPS	SET THREE WEIGHT/REPS

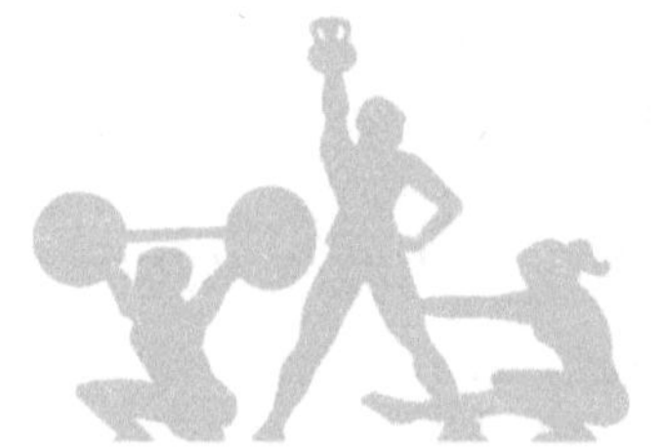

Name: ....

Date: ....

Time: ....

Warm-Up

ACTIVITY	TIME/REPS	DONE

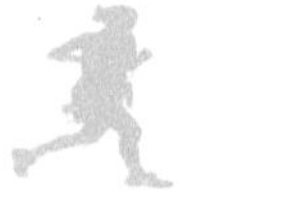 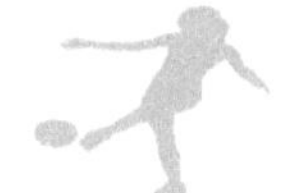 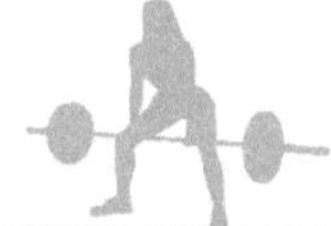 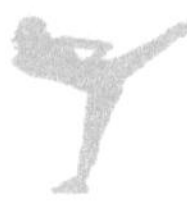 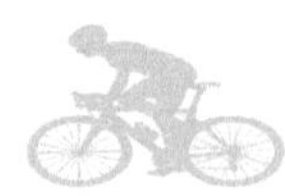

Cardio

ACTIVITY	DISTANCE	TIME	DONE

Weight Training

EXERCISE	SET ONE WEIGHT/REPS	SET TWO WEIGHT/REPS	SET THREE WEIGHT/REPS

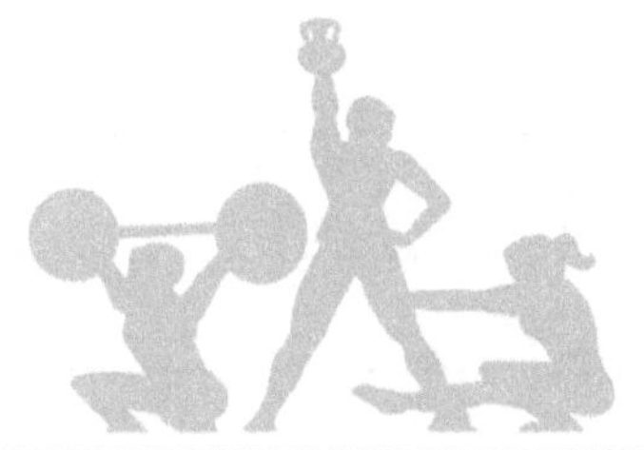

Name: ....

Date: ....

Time: ....

Warm-Up

ACTIVITY	TIME/REPS	DONE

 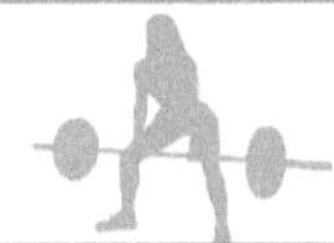 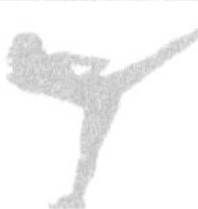 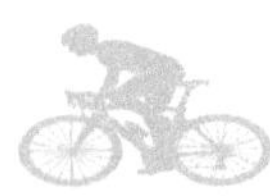

Cardio

ACTIVITY	DISTANCE	TIME	DONE

Weight Training

EXERCISE	SET ONE WEIGHT/REPS	SET TWO WEIGHT/REPS	SET THREE WEIGHT/REPS

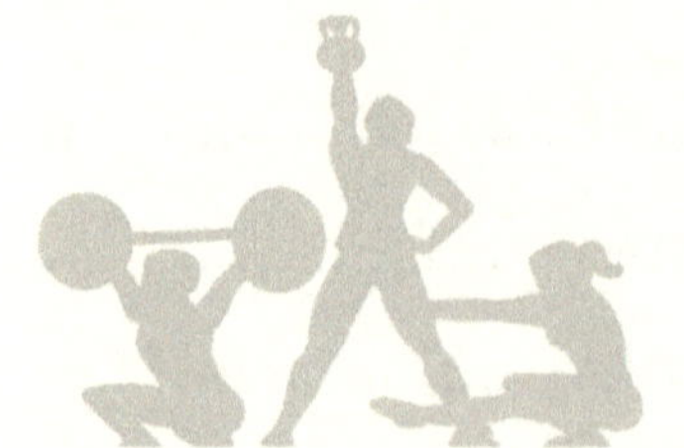

Name: ....

Date: ....

Time: ....

Warm-Up

ACTIVITY	TIME/REPS	DONE

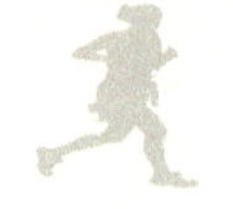 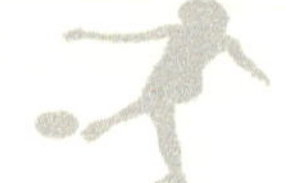 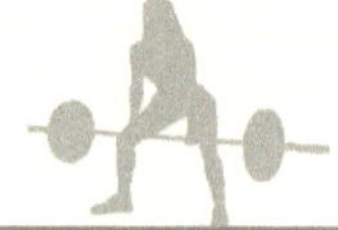 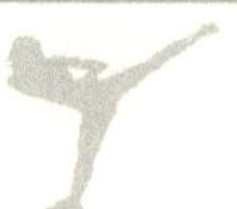 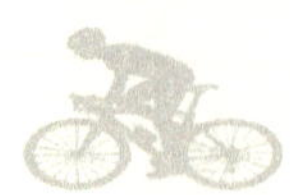

Cardio

ACTIVITY	DISTANCE	TIME	DONE

Weight Training

EXERCISE	SET ONE WEIGHT/REPS	SET TWO WEIGHT/REPS	SET THREE WEIGHT/REPS

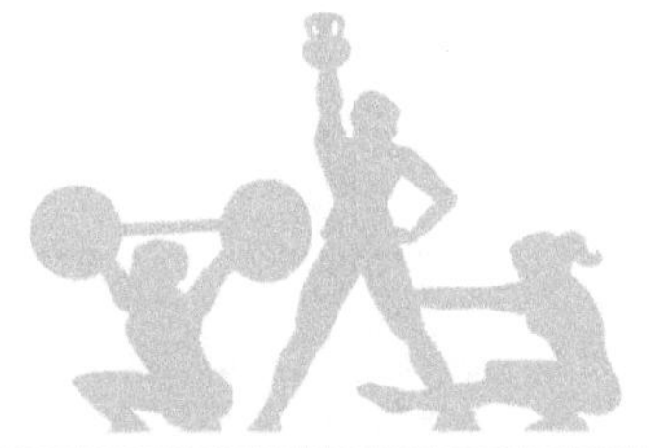

Name: ……………………………..

Date: ……………………………..

Time: ……………………………..

Warm-Up

ACTIVITY	TIME/REPS	DONE

 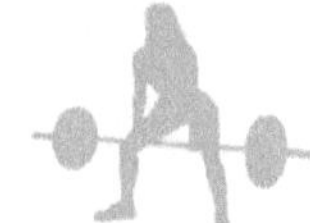 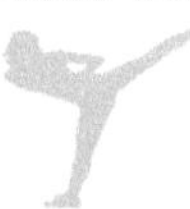 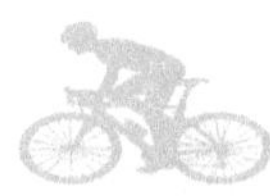

Cardio

ACTIVITY	DISTANCE	TIME	DONE

Weight Training

EXERCISE	SET ONE WEIGHT/REPS	SET TWO WEIGHT/REPS	SET THREE WEIGHT/REPS

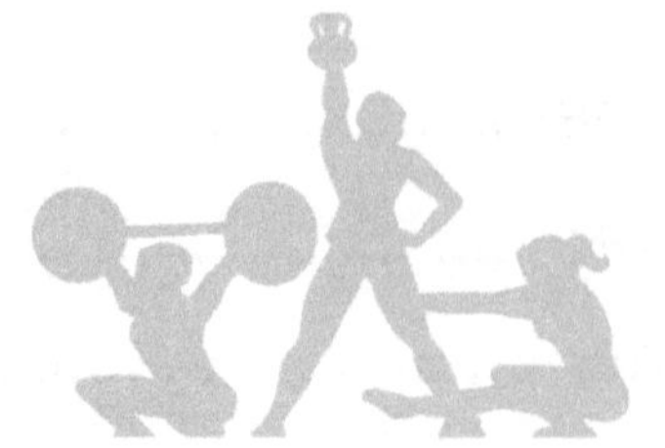

Name: ....

Date: ....

Time: ....

Warm-Up

ACTIVITY	TIME/REPS	DONE

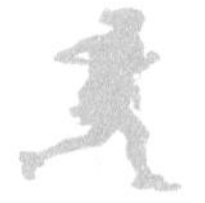 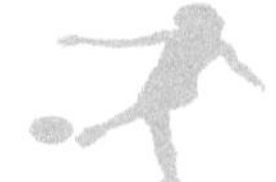 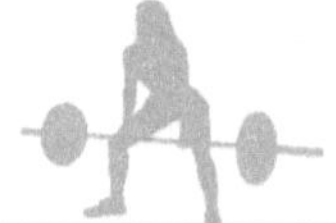 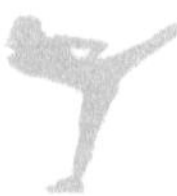 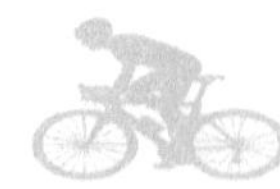

Cardio

ACTIVITY	DISTANCE	TIME	DONE

Weight Training

EXERCISE	SET ONE WEIGHT/REPS	SET TWO WEIGHT/REPS	SET THREE WEIGHT/REPS

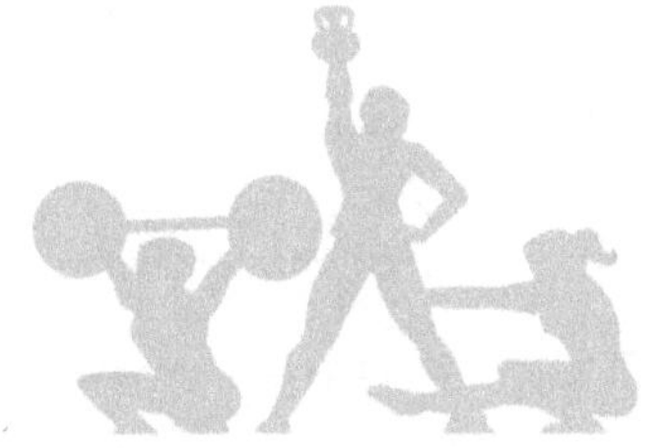

Name: …………………………

Date: …………………………

Time: …………………………

Warm-Up

ACTIVITY	TIME/REPS	DONE

 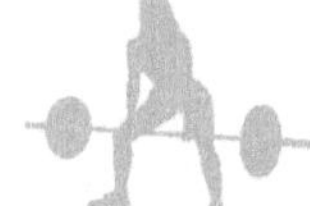 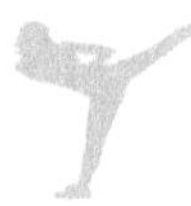 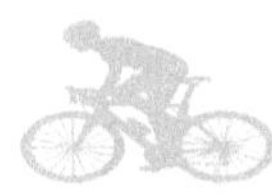

Cardio

ACTIVITY	DISTANCE	TIME	DONE

Weight Training

EXERCISE	SET ONE WEIGHT/REPS	SET TWO WEIGHT/REPS	SET THREE WEIGHT/REPS

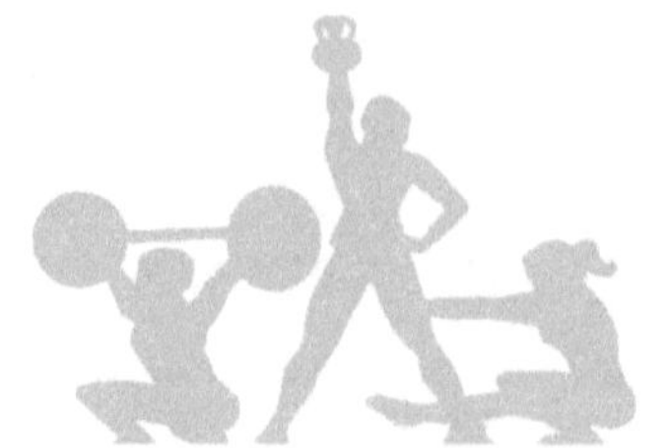

Warm-Up

ACTIVITY	TIME/REPS	DONE

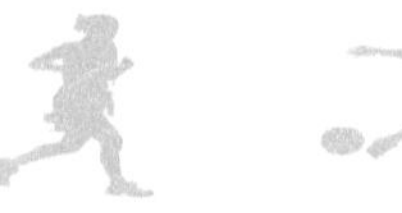 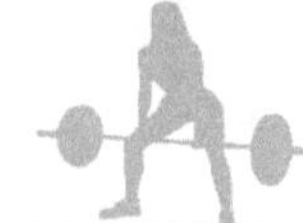 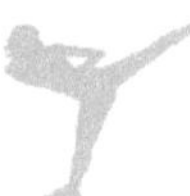 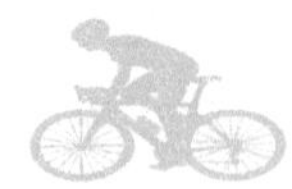

Cardio

ACTIVITY	DISTANCE	TIME	DONE

Weight Training

EXERCISE	SET ONE WEIGHT/REPS	SET TWO WEIGHT/REPS	SET THREE WEIGHT/REPS

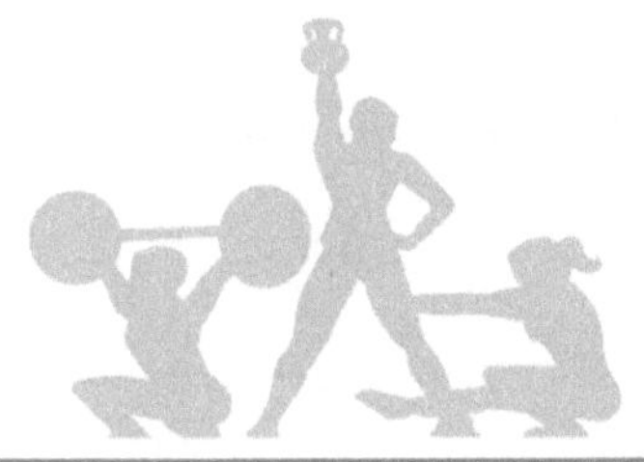

Name: ....

Date: ....

Time: ....

Warm-Up

ACTIVITY	TIME/REPS	DONE

 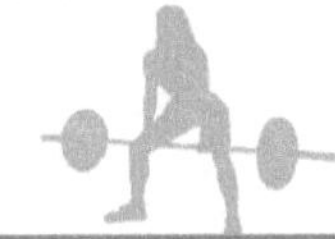 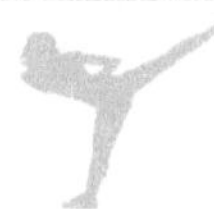 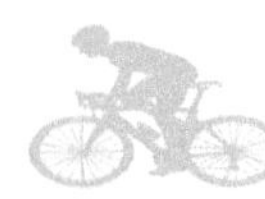

Cardio

ACTIVITY	DISTANCE	TIME	DONE

Weight Training

EXERCISE	SET ONE WEIGHT/REPS	SET TWO WEIGHT/REPS	SET THREE WEIGHT/REPS

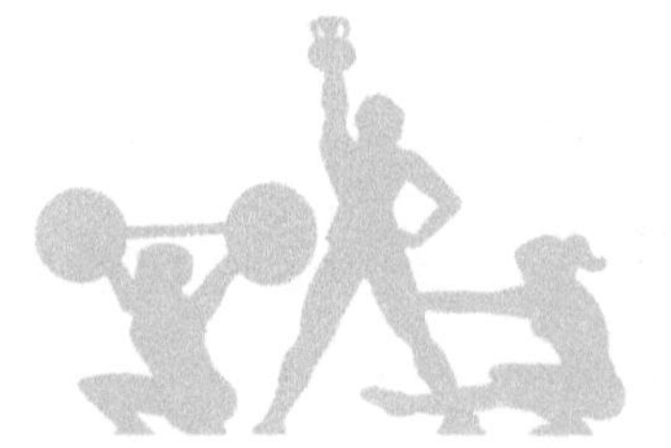

Name: ....

Date: ....

Time: ....

Warm-Up

ACTIVITY	TIME/REPS	DONE

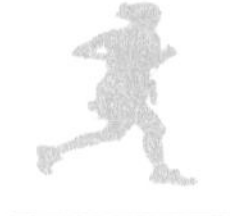 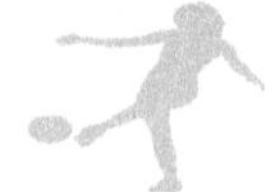 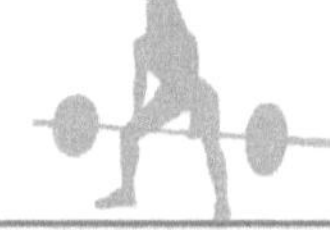 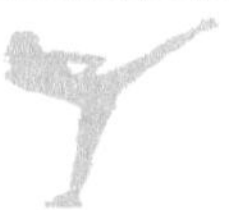 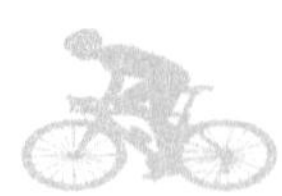

Cardio

ACTIVITY	DISTANCE	TIME	DONE

Weight Training

EXERCISE	SET ONE WEIGHT/REPS	SET TWO WEIGHT/REPS	SET THREE WEIGHT/REPS

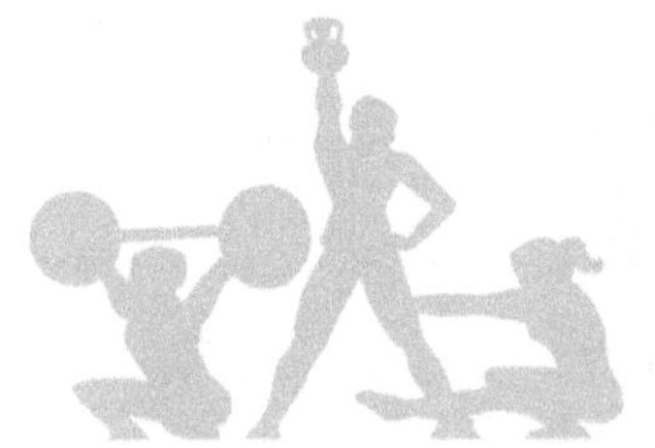

Name: ....

Date: ....

Time: ....

Warm-Up

ACTIVITY	TIME/REPS	DONE

 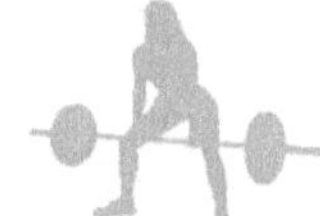 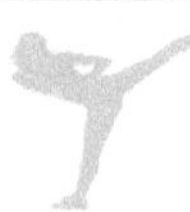 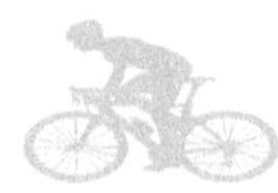

Cardio

ACTIVITY	DISTANCE	TIME	DONE

Weight Training

EXERCISE	SET ONE WEIGHT/REPS	SET TWO WEIGHT/REPS	SET THREE WEIGHT/REPS

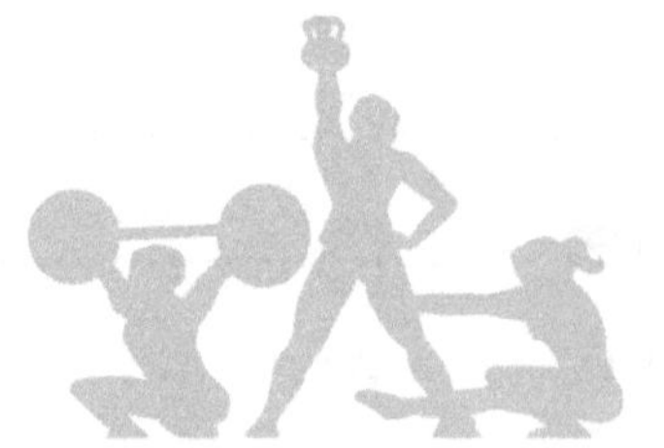

Name: ....

Date: ....

Time: ....

Warm-Up

ACTIVITY	TIME/REPS	DONE

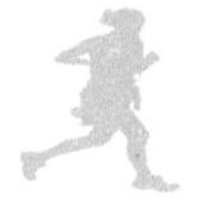 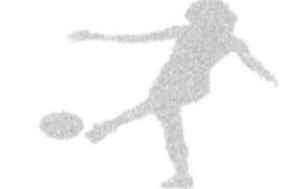 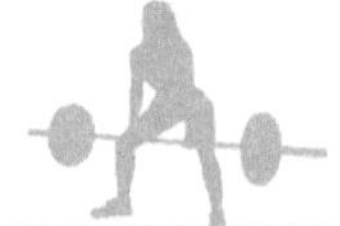 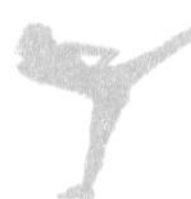 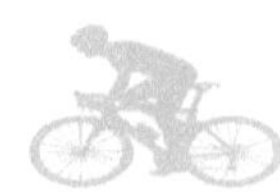

Cardio

ACTIVITY	DISTANCE	TIME	DONE

Weight Training

EXERCISE	SET ONE WEIGHT/REPS	SET TWO WEIGHT/REPS	SET THREE WEIGHT/REPS

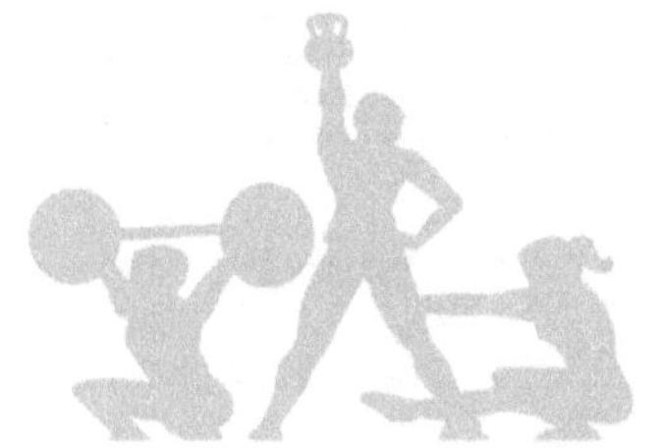

Warm-Up

ACTIVITY	TIME/REPS	DONE

 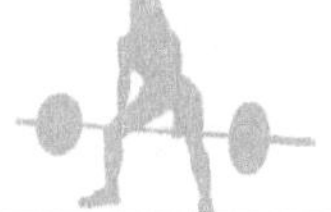 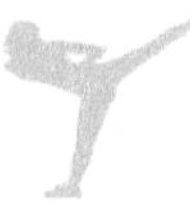 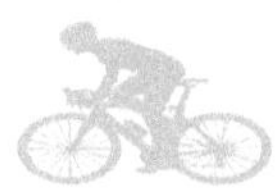

Cardio

ACTIVITY	DISTANCE	TIME	DONE

Weight Training

EXERCISE	SET ONE WEIGHT/REPS	SET TWO WEIGHT/REPS	SET THREE WEIGHT/REPS

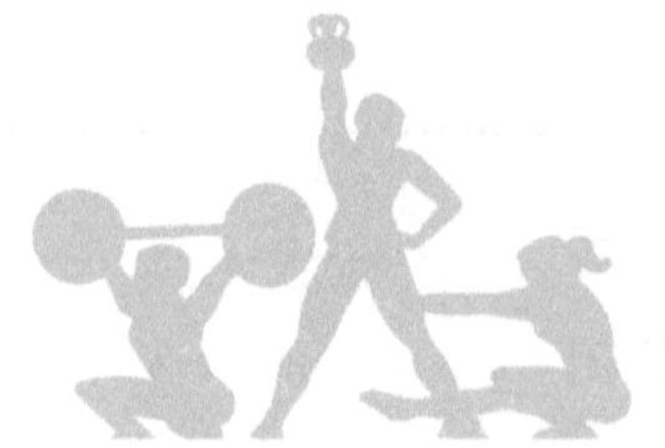

Name: ....

Date: ....

Time: ....

Warm-Up

ACTIVITY	TIME/REPS	DONE

 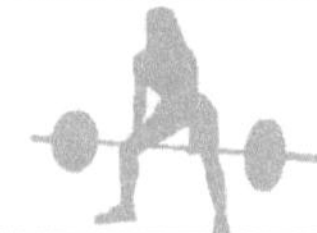 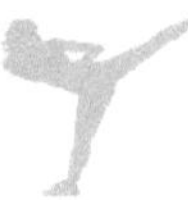 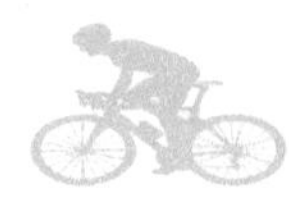

Cardio

ACTIVITY	DISTANCE	TIME	DONE

Weight Training

EXERCISE	SET ONE WEIGHT/REPS	SET TWO WEIGHT/REPS	SET THREE WEIGHT/REPS

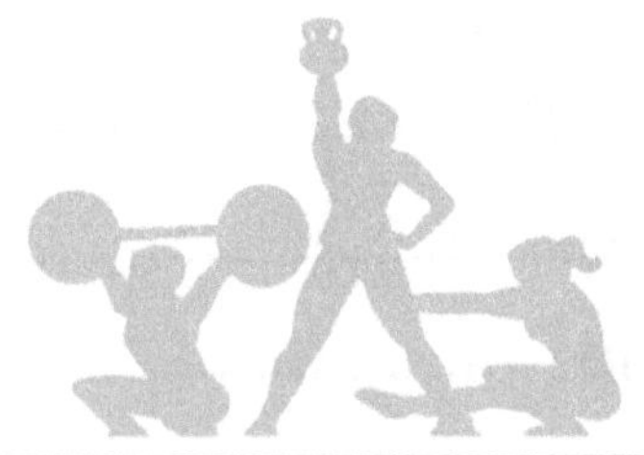

Name: ....

Date: ....

Time: ....

Warm-Up

ACTIVITY	TIME/REPS	DONE

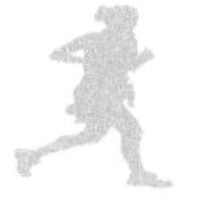 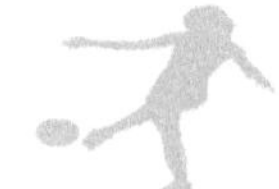 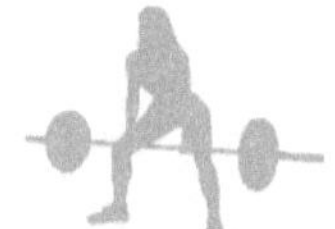 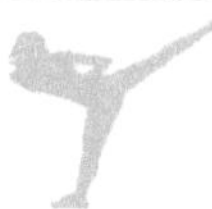 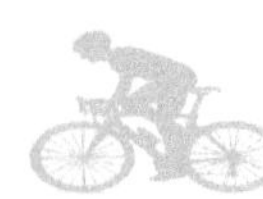

Cardio

ACTIVITY	DISTANCE	TIME	DONE

Weight Training

EXERCISE	SET ONE WEIGHT/REPS	SET TWO WEIGHT/REPS	SET THREE WEIGHT/REPS

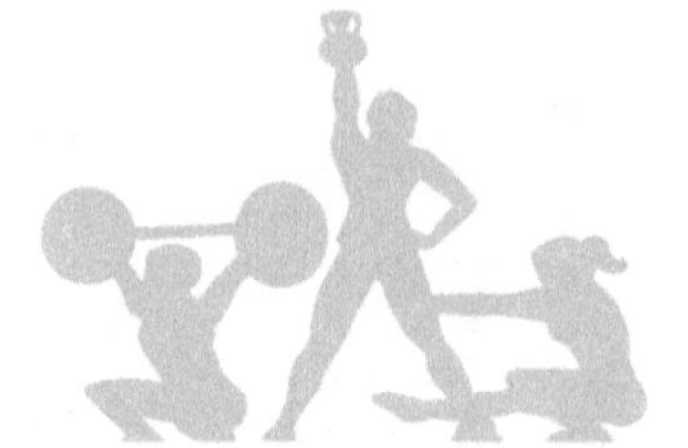

Name: ....

Date: ....

Time: ....

Warm-Up

ACTIVITY	TIME/REPS	DONE

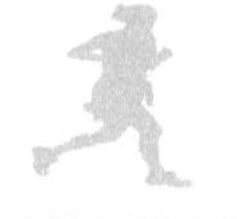 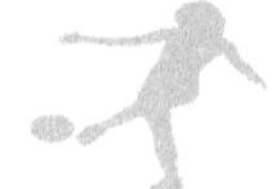 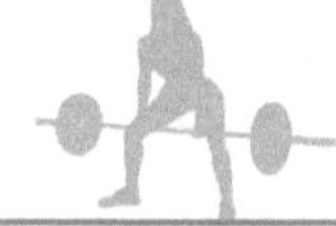 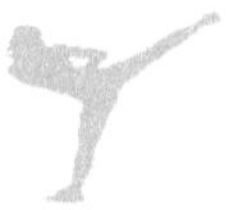 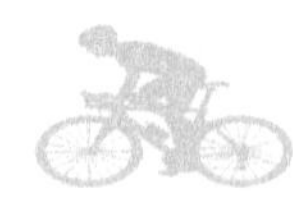

Cardio

ACTIVITY	DISTANCE	TIME	DONE

Weight Training

EXERCISE	SET ONE WEIGHT/REPS	SET TWO WEIGHT/REPS	SET THREE WEIGHT/REPS

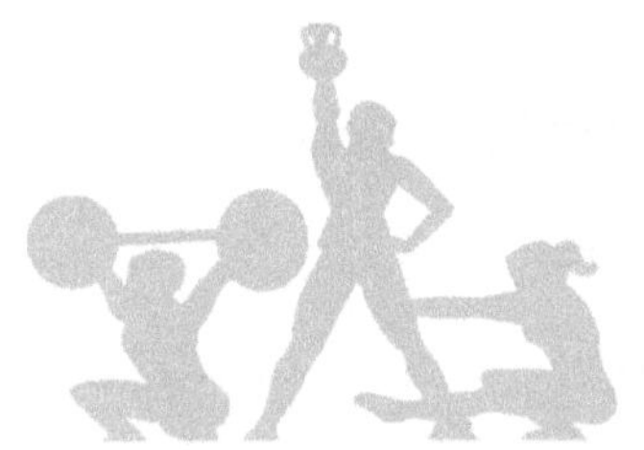

Name: ....

Date: ....

Time: ....

Warm-Up

ACTIVITY	TIME/REPS	DONE

 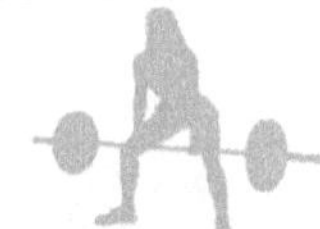 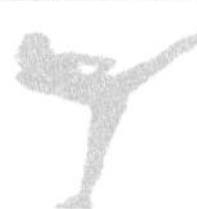 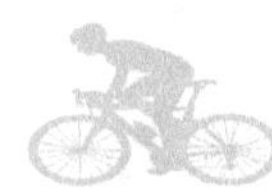

Cardio

ACTIVITY	DISTANCE	TIME	DONE

Weight Training

EXERCISE	SET ONE WEIGHT/REPS	SET TWO WEIGHT/REPS	SET THREE WEIGHT/REPS

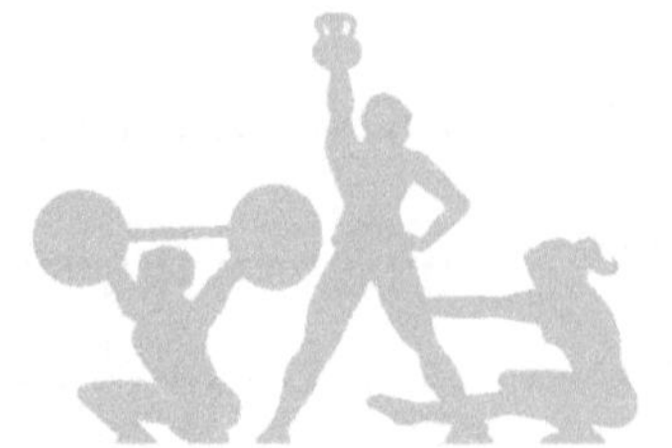

Name: ....

Date: ....

Time: ....

Warm-Up

ACTIVITY	TIME/REPS	DONE

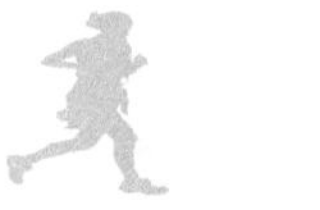 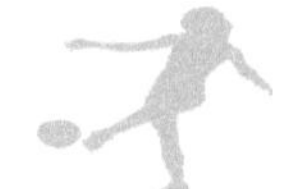 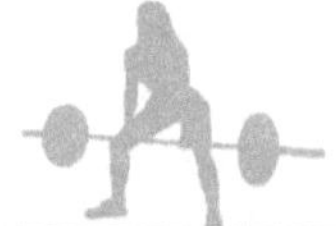 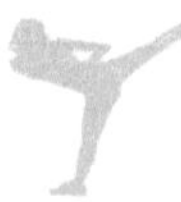 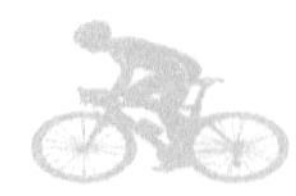

Cardio

ACTIVITY	DISTANCE	TIME	DONE

Weight Training

EXERCISE	SET ONE WEIGHT/REPS	SET TWO WEIGHT/REPS	SET THREE WEIGHT/REPS

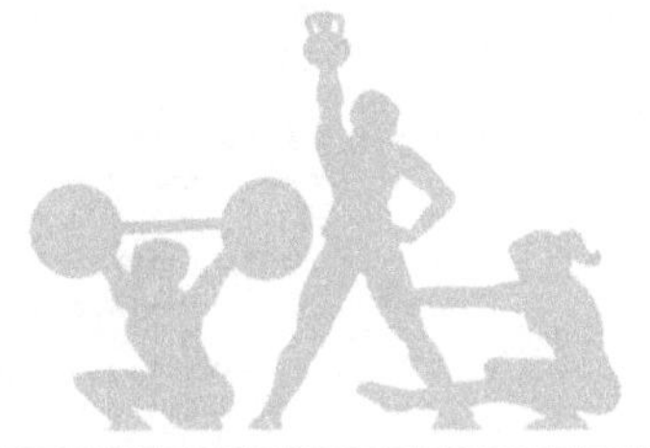

Warm-Up

ACTIVITY	TIME/REPS	DONE

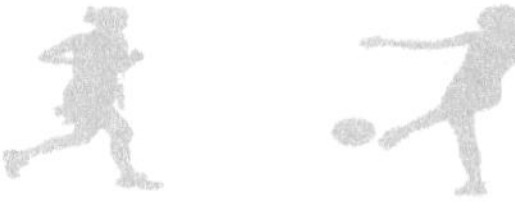 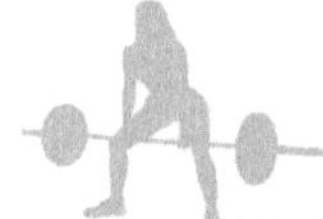 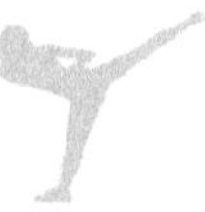 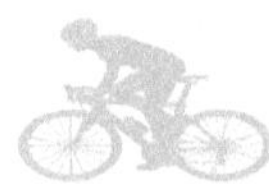

Cardio

ACTIVITY	DISTANCE	TIME	DONE

Weight Training

EXERCISE	SET ONE WEIGHT/REPS	SET TWO WEIGHT/REPS	SET THREE WEIGHT/REPS

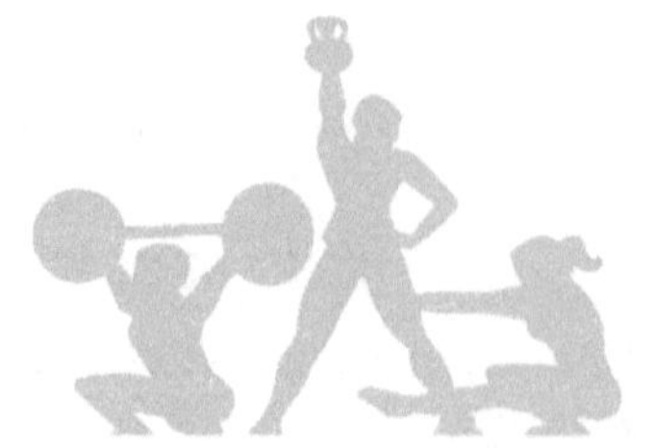

Name: ....

Date: ....

Time: ....

Warm-Up

ACTIVITY	TIME/REPS	DONE

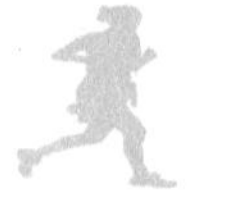 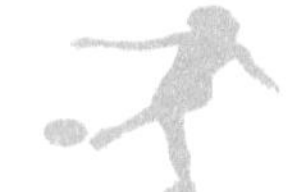 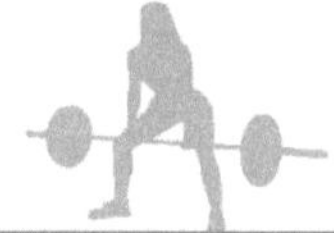 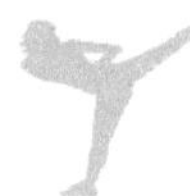 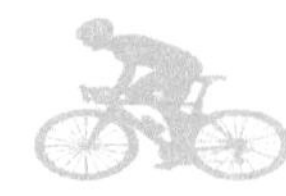

Cardio

ACTIVITY	DISTANCE	TIME	DONE

Weight Training

EXERCISE	SET ONE WEIGHT/REPS	SET TWO WEIGHT/REPS	SET THREE WEIGHT/REPS

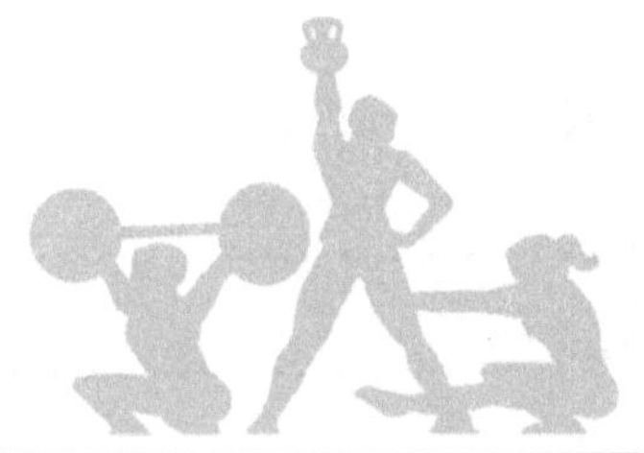

Name: ....

Date: ....

Time: ....

Warm-Up

ACTIVITY	TIME/REPS	DONE

  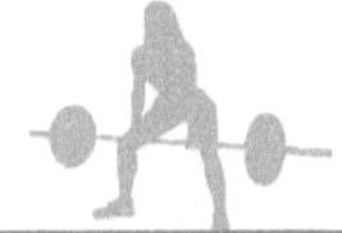 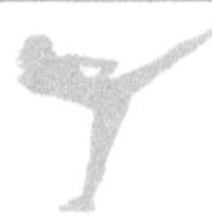 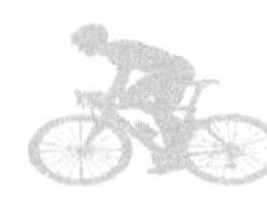

Cardio

ACTIVITY	DISTANCE	TIME	DONE

Weight Training

EXERCISE	SET ONE WEIGHT/REPS	SET TWO WEIGHT/REPS	SET THREE WEIGHT/REPS

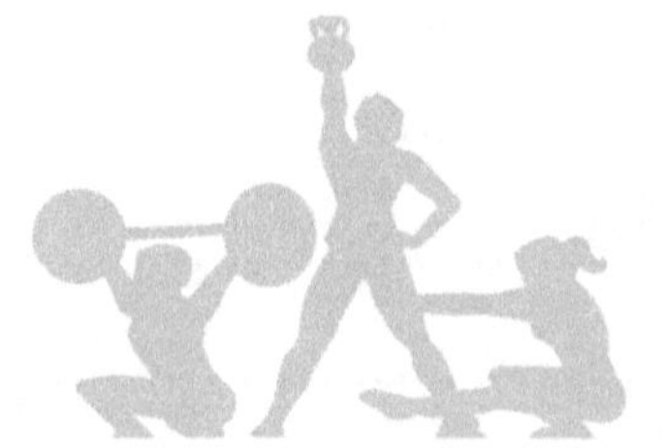

Name: ....

Date: ....

Time: ....

Warm-Up

ACTIVITY	TIME/REPS	DONE

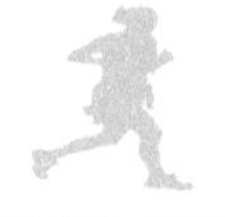 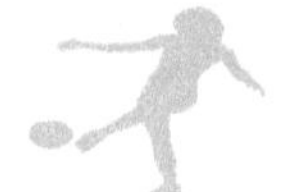 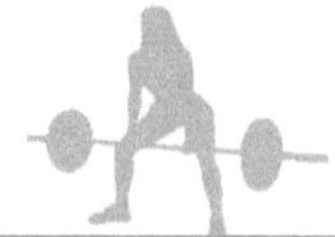 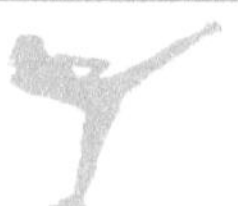 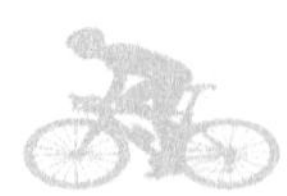

Cardio

ACTIVITY	DISTANCE	TIME	DONE

Weight Training

EXERCISE	SET ONE WEIGHT/REPS	SET TWO WEIGHT/REPS	SET THREE WEIGHT/REPS

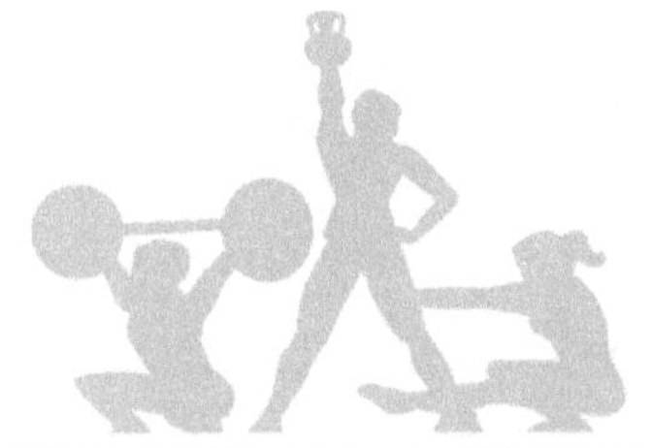

Name: ……………………………

Date: ……………………………

Time: ……………………………

Warm-Up

ACTIVITY	TIME/REPS	DONE

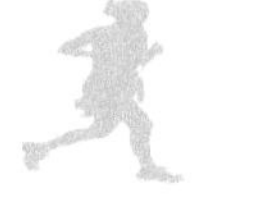 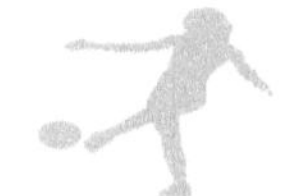 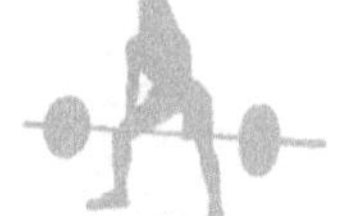 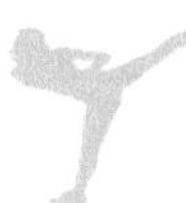 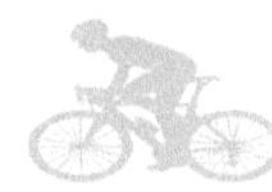

Cardio

ACTIVITY	DISTANCE	TIME	DONE

Weight Training

EXERCISE	SET ONE WEIGHT/REPS	SET TWO WEIGHT/REPS	SET THREE WEIGHT/REPS

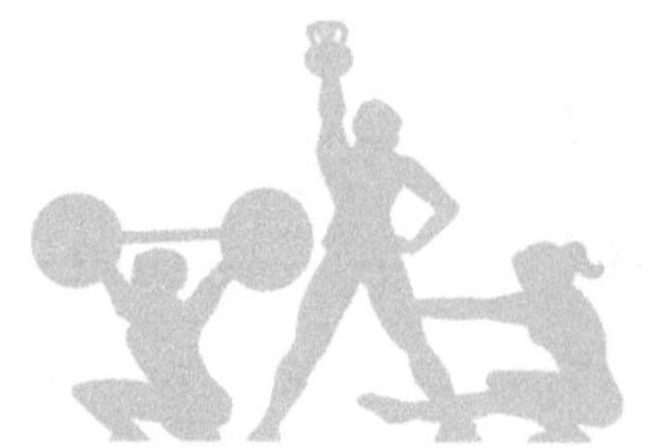

Name: ....

Date: ....

Time: ....

Warm-Up

ACTIVITY	TIME/REPS	DONE

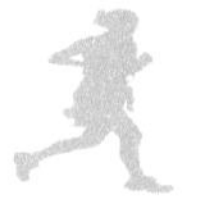 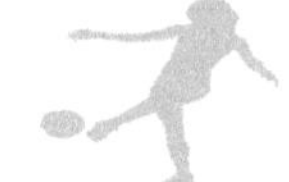 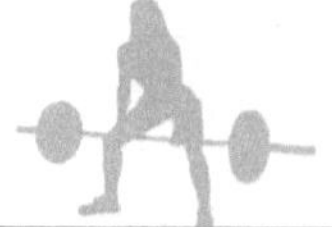 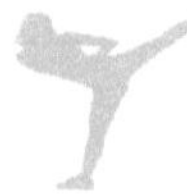 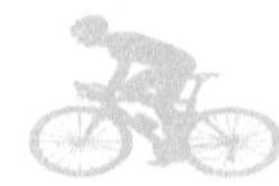

Cardio

ACTIVITY	DISTANCE	TIME	DONE

Weight Training

EXERCISE	SET ONE WEIGHT/REPS	SET TWO WEIGHT/REPS	SET THREE WEIGHT/REPS

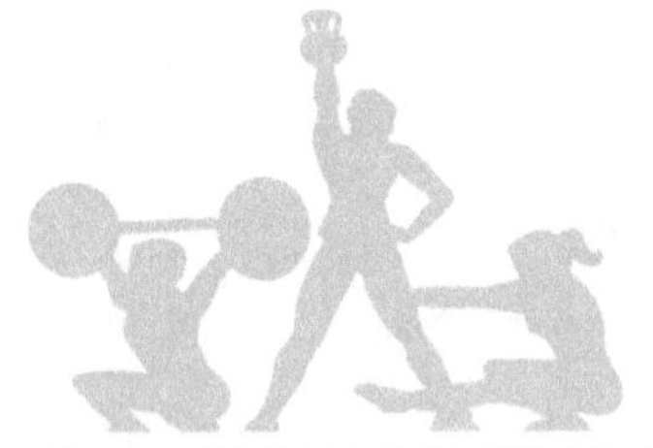

Name: ……………………………

Date: ……………………………

Time: ……………………………

Warm-Up

ACTIVITY	TIME/REPS	DONE

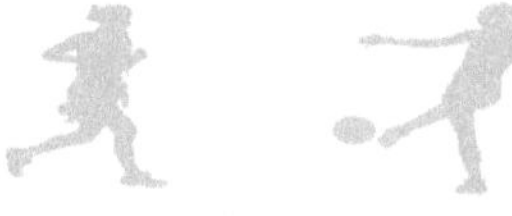  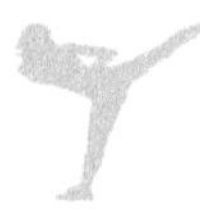 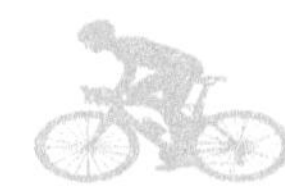

Cardio

ACTIVITY	DISTANCE	TIME	DONE

Weight Training

EXERCISE	SET ONE WEIGHT/REPS	SET TWO WEIGHT/REPS	SET THREE WEIGHT/REPS

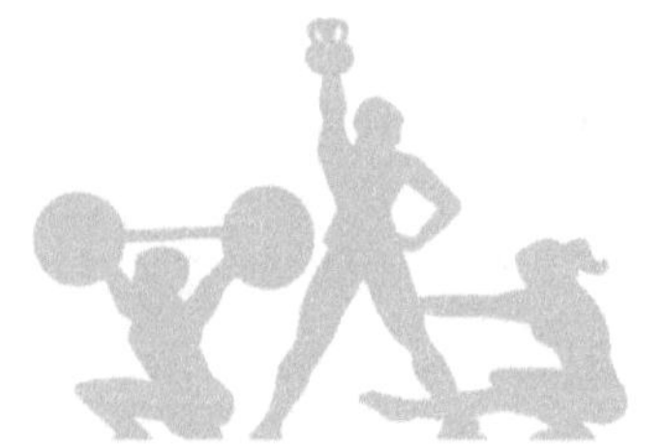

Name: ....

Date: ....

Time: ....

Warm-Up

ACTIVITY	TIME/REPS	DONE

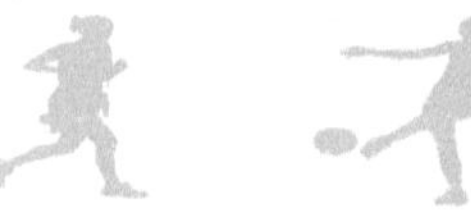 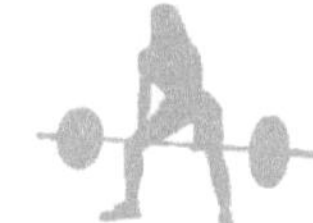 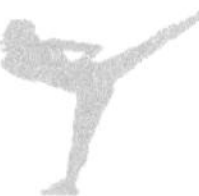 

Cardio

ACTIVITY	DISTANCE	TIME	DONE

Weight Training

EXERCISE	SET ONE WEIGHT/REPS	SET TWO WEIGHT/REPS	SET THREE WEIGHT/REPS

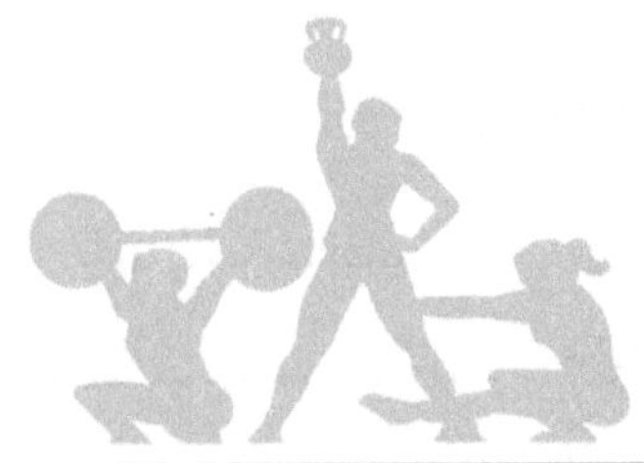

Name: ……………………………

Date: ……………………………

Time: ……………………………

Warm-Up

ACTIVITY	TIME/REPS	DONE

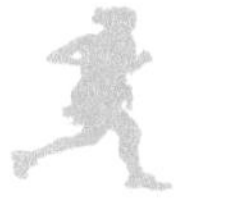 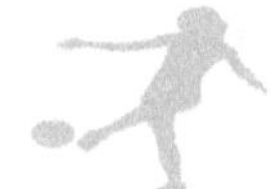 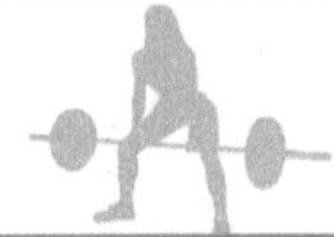 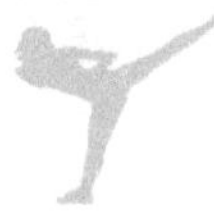 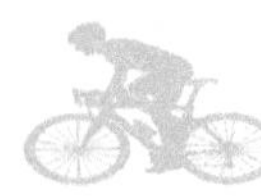

Cardio

ACTIVITY	DISTANCE	TIME	DONE

Weight Training

EXERCISE	SET ONE WEIGHT/REPS	SET TWO WEIGHT/REPS	SET THREE WEIGHT/REPS

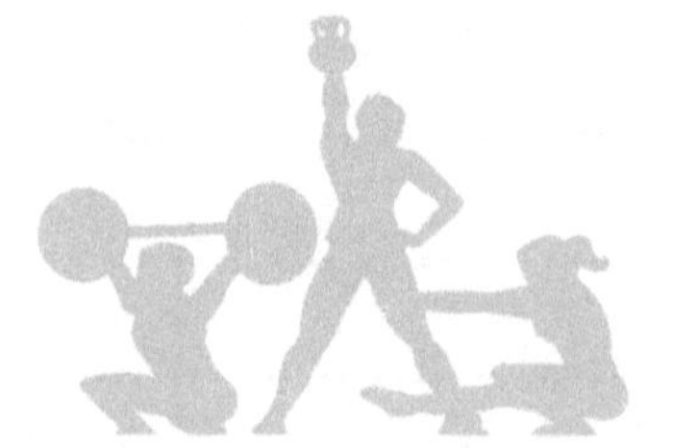

Warm-Up

ACTIVITY	TIME/REPS	DONE

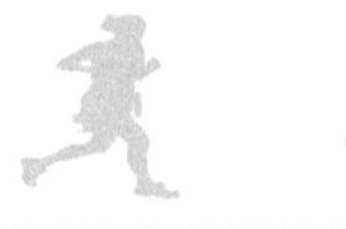   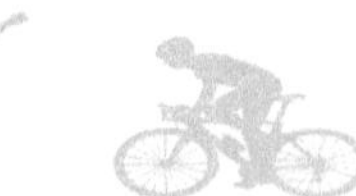

Cardio

ACTIVITY	DISTANCE	TIME	DONE

Weight Training

EXERCISE	SET ONE WEIGHT/REPS	SET TWO WEIGHT/REPS	SET THREE WEIGHT/REPS

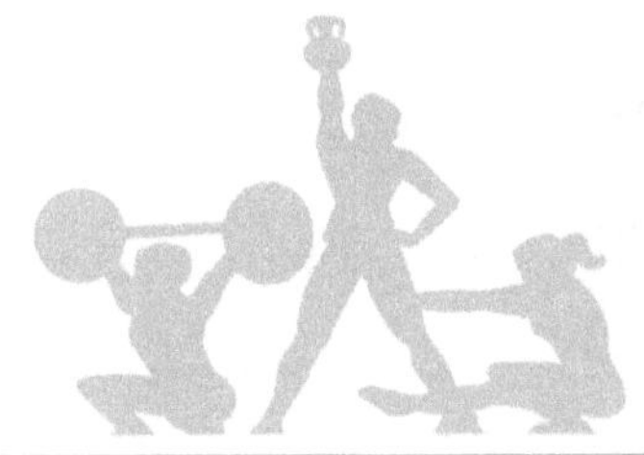

Name: ....

Date: ....

Time: ....

Warm-Up

ACTIVITY	TIME/REPS	DONE

 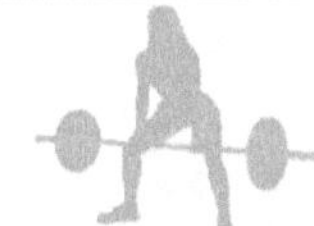 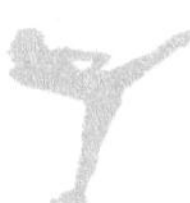 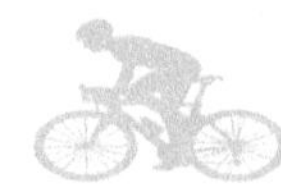

Cardio

ACTIVITY	DISTANCE	TIME	DONE

Weight Training

EXERCISE	SET ONE WEIGHT/REPS	SET TWO WEIGHT/REPS	SET THREE WEIGHT/REPS

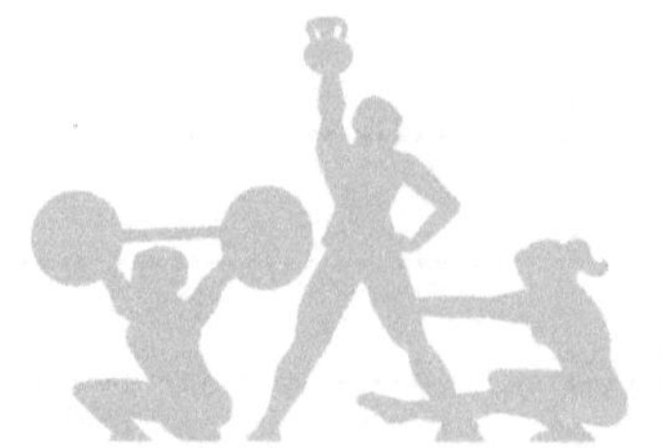

Name: ....

Date: ....

Time: ....

Warm-Up

ACTIVITY	TIME/REPS	DONE

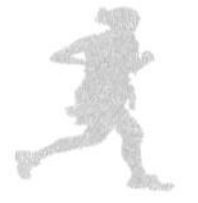  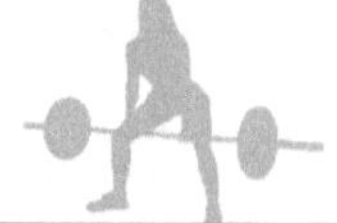 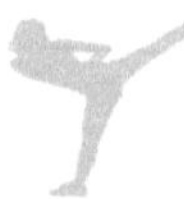 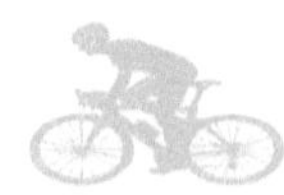

Cardio

ACTIVITY	DISTANCE	TIME	DONE

Weight Training

EXERCISE	SET ONE WEIGHT/REPS	SET TWO WEIGHT/REPS	SET THREE WEIGHT/REPS

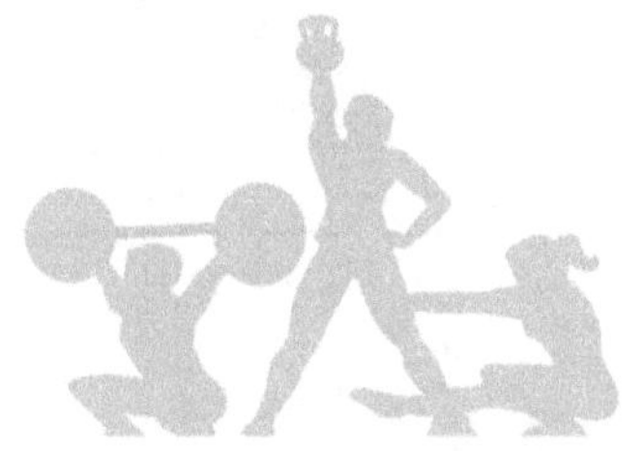

Name: ....

Date: ....

Time: ....

Warm-Up

ACTIVITY	TIME/REPS	DONE

 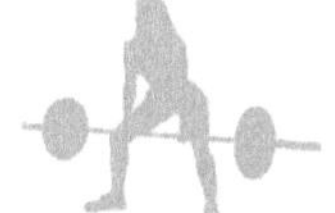 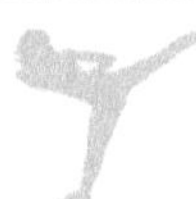 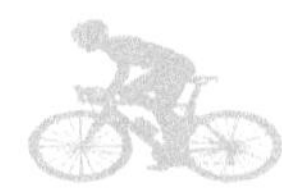

Cardio

ACTIVITY	DISTANCE	TIME	DONE

Weight Training

EXERCISE	SET ONE WEIGHT/REPS	SET TWO WEIGHT/REPS	SET THREE WEIGHT/REPS

Weekly Weight Tracker

Name.................................
Starting Weight................
Target Weight...................

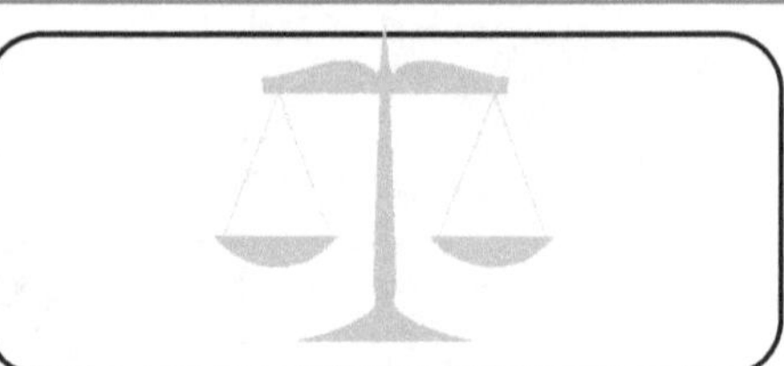

DATE	CURRENT WEIGHT	WEIGHT LOST	WEIGHT GAINED

Weekly Weight Tracker

Name..................................

Starting Weight.................

Target Weight...................

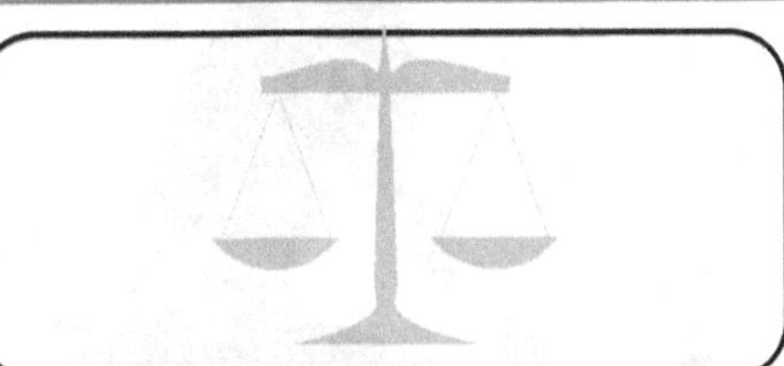

DATE	CURRENT WEIGHT	WEIGHT LOST	WEIGHT GAINED

NOTES